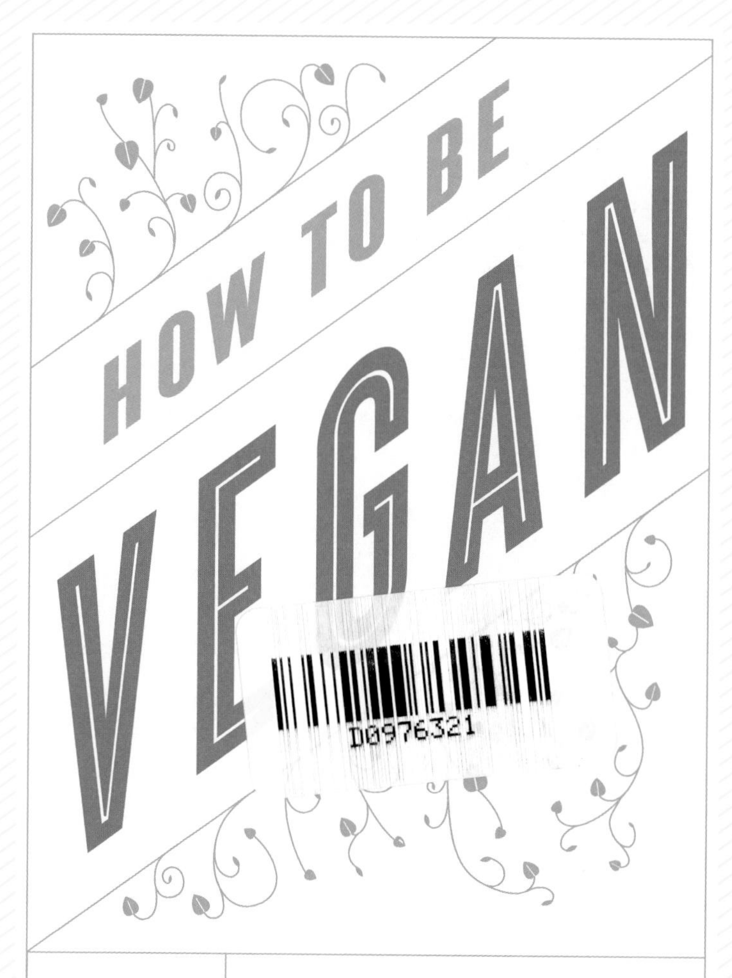

HOW TO BE VEGAN

ELIZABETH CASTORIA

With recipes by
ROBIN ROBERTSON

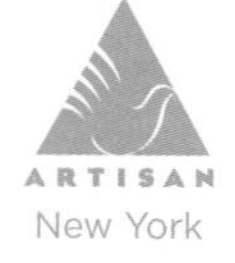

ARTISAN
New York

Published by Artisan
A division of Workman Publishing Company, Inc.
225 Varick Street
New York, NY 10014-4381
artisanbooks.com

Published simultaneously in Canada by Thomas Allen & Son, Limited

---

Library of Congress Cataloging-in-Publication Data

Castoria, Elizabeth.
How to be vegan / Elizabeth Castoria ; with recipes by Robin Robertson.
pages cm
Includes index.
ISBN 978-1-57965-555-6
1. Vegan cooking. I. Robertson, Robin (Robin G.). II. Title.
TX837.C348 2014
641.5'636—dc23 2013029978

Design & Illustration by Paul Kepple & Ralph Geroni at Headcase Design

Printed in the United States
First printing, March 2014
10 9 8 7 6 5 4 3 2 1

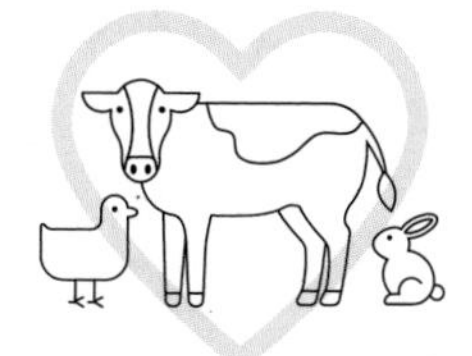

To the curious and for the animals

CONTENTS

Let's Start!

Bravo! You're considering trying out this whole plant-based-eating idea. That is flat-out wonderful, and there's some good news to start you on your way: it's a little-known secret that going vegan is the easiest self-help strategy in the history of the world. To be vegan, you don't have to do anything; you just have to *not* do one thing. Going vegan is a blissfully simple one-step process. Ready? Here it is: stop buying animal products. Done. Voilà. *Finito.* And kudos, you are now a freshly minted vegan, fully equipped with a new vegan scent and everything.

Though straightforward, this single step can be taken at various paces for various people. For some, it could take a good ten years of dabbling before they decide to go vegan full throttle. For others, it takes about as long as it will to read to the end of this sentence. But here's the thing: in merely thinking about maybe someday (possibly today, for

"Life isn't about finding yourself.
Life is about creating yourself."

—GEORGE BERNARD SHAW

type A personalities) trying out veganism, you've already done something great. You've already entertained the possibility that this lifestyle might have merit, and being open to that concept is a victory in itself.

The reasons to give veganism a shot are legion—from helping save the planet to being kind to animals to reducing your chances of dying from a heart attack. You might even have rolled all these lofty and admirable goals into one, or, as in my case about a million years ago, you might be trying to impress a devilishly cute seventeen-year-old skater who is, like, really deep. (Note: skaters come and go, but they can have a lasting effect!)

Whatever your reasons for ditching meat and dairy, fantastic. I hope you'll find that this book helps to demystify, destigmatize, and uncomplicate veganism. This book is by no means an encyclopedia; there are intricacies and tangential issues that we simply won't go into here. Think of the book as a springboard. Vegan 101. Maybe something will catch your eye and you'll want to dig deeper (Resources start on page 214). Maybe you're looking for a really great pancake recipe (recipes await you on page 149). Maybe you're just looking to impress the cute vegan you always see at the gym and need some tips on how to woo appropriately. From getting all the nutrients a healthy body needs to ridding your closet of animal cruelty, we'll go over the basics of exactly how to live vegan. Here we go!

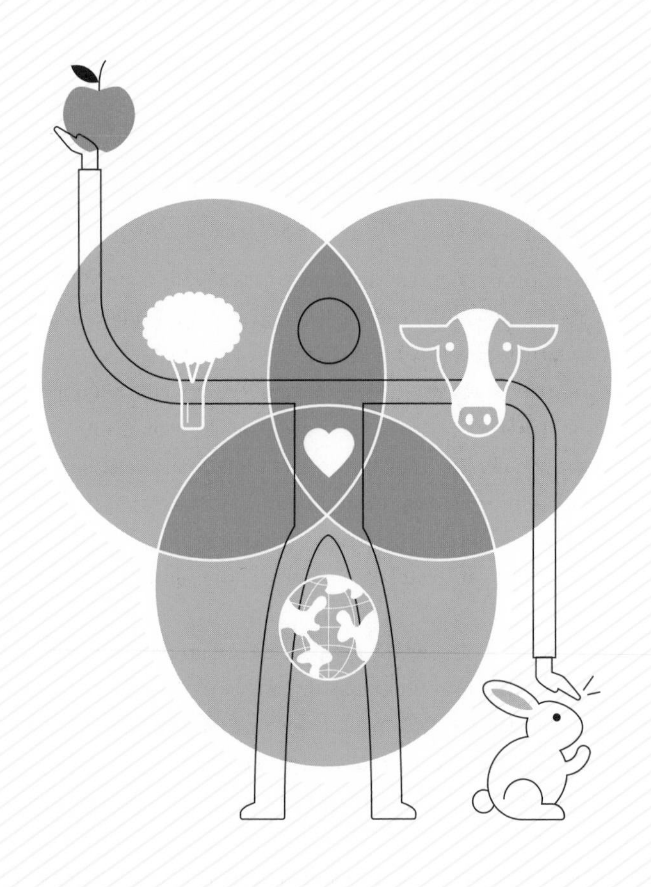

1

THE BASICS

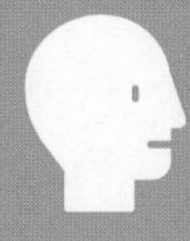

HERE'S THE 4-1-1

"The perfect is the enemy of the good."

—VOLTAIRE

There are roughly 800 zillion great reasons to go vegan. There is also one thing we should get straight right away, just so there isn't any confusion about it later on. It's one of the world's best-kept secrets: it is impossible to be 100 percent vegan, meaning that it is impossible to live in the world and avoid coming into contact with animal products altogether. Your precious energy and time are better spent making the changes that will have the biggest impact. That's right—what you do has a direct effect on the state of the world. We can create the kind of world we want to live in with the choices we make, which, frankly, is maybe the most exciting realization of all time.

Does cutting eggs out of your diet confer incredible health benefits, improve the state of the environment, and eliminate a great deal of animal suffering? Yes. Does interrogating the eighteen-year-old waiter who makes minimum wage and really just wants to go home after working a double shift about whether the pots in the kitchen have ever touched meat do the same things? No. There are no merit badges for being the most vegan person in the room, no secret handshakes for people who've been vegan the longest. Trying out this lifestyle is an opportunity to think about our daily choices in a new, exciting way, not a route to personal perfection.

Defining the Ways We Eat

There's a pretty straightforward definition of being a vegan: someone who does not consume animal products. But what about the ovo-lacto-pesca-graina-fruita-tarians you hear about these days? With so many different kinds of eaters out there, where do vegans fit in to the food chain? Here's a simple breakdown.

VEGANS: People who don't eat, wear, or use animal products.

VEGETARIANS: People who don't eat meat (that means no chicken or fish either—those aren't plants!) but do eat eggs and dairy.

OVO-LACTO VEGETARIANS: This is basically just the 1970s term for a vegetarian. You might hear this used in contrast to a "pure vegetarian," which means a vegan. *Ovo* means "eggs," and *lacto* means "milk," so sometimes people will identify themselves as ovo vegetarians (meaning they do eat eggs but don't consume dairy), or lacto vegetarians (vice versa).

PESCATARIANS: Those who eat eggs, milk, and fish but not chicken, pork, beef, or other land animals.

FLEXITARIANS: Flexitarians eat vegan or vegetarian some of the time, as a conscious effort (in comparison to, say, someone who happens to eat a salad for lunch without considering at all the fact that the salad was a choice).

MEAT REDUCERS: Much like flexitarians, these people want to cut down on the amount of meat they consume and may conscientiously opt for plant-based meals.

RAW-FOODISTS: Those who eat uncooked food and usually eat a mostly, if not wholly, vegan diet. There are raw-foodists who drink raw milk (and a few who eat raw meat), so it's not safe to assume that someone on a raw diet is also vegan or vice versa.

DIETARY DIFFERENCES, AT A GLANCE

	plants	eggs	cheese	fish	steak
VEGAN	what they eat	what they don't eat	what they don't eat	what they don't eat	what they don't eat
VEGETARIAN	what they eat	what they eat	what they eat	what they don't eat	what they don't eat
PESCATARIAN	what they eat	what they eat	what they eat	what they eat	what they don't eat
FLEXITARIAN	what they eat	what they eat	what they eat	what they eat	what they eat
MEAT REDUCER	what they eat	what they eat	what they eat	what they eat	what they eat
OMNIVORE	what they eat	what they eat	what they eat	what they eat	what they eat

● what they eat ● what they don't eat

LEVEL-FIVE VEGANS: This was just a really clever joke on *The Simpsons,* during the episode "Lisa the Tree Hugger." A character quips, "I'm a level-five vegan—I won't eat anything that casts a shadow."

How Does One Go About Being Vegan?

For some people, watching five seconds of video footage from a factory farm will do the trick; others will start by cutting out certain products and then gradually expand that list until they're fully vegan. There are a few different approaches to going vegan. Mark Bittman, a columnist for *The New York Times,* released a cookbook called *VB6,* which stands for "vegan before 6:00 P.M." After his doctor recommended that he adopt a plant-based diet to improve his health, Bittman decided that he'd be totally vegan during the day and then eat whatever he felt like for dinner. Kathy Freston, a noted self-help author, penned *The Lean,* which encourages readers to "lean in" to veganism by including more plants in their diets and gradually filling up until there's no room for the steak frites. Across the country, schools, hospitals, city governments, and businesses have adopted Meatless Mondays, which is just what it sounds like: not eating meat on Monday in an effort to eat a more plant-rich diet. But finding a method of going vegan that works for you and makes you feel good is much more important than adhering to a strict set of rules.

Most people who are interested in a vegan lifestyle seem to get a little taste at some point, and then go further and further with it as time goes on. Maybe you stop buying animal products altogether on your

FIVE START-HERE BOOKS

These easy beginner books help explain how and why veganism is fantastic for you, the planet, and animals. (Note that these are not cookbooks; find a list of those on page 214.)

- *Eating Animals*, by Jonathan Safran Foer
- *The Face on Your Plate*, by Jeffrey Moussaieff Masson
- *Finding Ultra*, by Rich Roll
- *The Lean*, by Kathy Freston
- *Mad Cowboy*, by Howard F. Lyman with Glen Merzer

next shopping trip, or maybe you start removing one animal-based food and replacing it with three plant foods per week. Maybe you eat totally vegan at home and then slowly begin to do so when you go out, too. One of the best ways to go about this is to plan your weekly menu (more on that in Chapter 6). Lining up an array of delicious dishes is sure to excite your imagination and taste buds!

A HANDY CHECKLIST

Why do you want to be vegan? (Check all that apply.)

- ◯ For my health
- ◯ Because I like animals
- ◯ Because I wouldn't want to work in a slaughterhouse
- ◯ Because I want to live my values
- ◯ To help the planet
- ◯ Because everyone else is doing it

Why Go Vegan?

People choose to munch plants for lots of reasons, but there are basically four big, overarching reasons: concern for personal health, concern for the environment, concern for animals, and concern for other people. Here's a snapshot of each of those.

PERSONAL HEALTH

Take this short quiz to determine whether health is among the reasons veganism might be important to you. Please answer the following questions yes or no, to the best of your knowledge:

1.	Do you enjoy going to parties, spruced up in your spiffiest duds, reveling in the company of good people, sipping delectable party drinks, and coming home exhausted after a night on the dance floor?	◯ Yes ◯ No
2.	Do you enjoy having friends with whom to throw said parties? Do you think those close to you might continue to enjoy your company for the foreseeable future?	◯ Yes ◯ No
3.	Do you enjoy sunshine, blossoming cherry trees, hugging puppies, reading books (if your answer here is no, thanks for making the extra effort!), traveling to new and exciting destinations, celebrating birthdays (yours or others'), or doing absolutely anything else that someone who is alive might conceivably enjoy?	◯ Yes ◯ No

If you answered yes to any of these questions, good news! Health is likely something that matters to you. Unequivocally, going vegan is one of the best things you can do for your health. The average man in the United States has a 50 percent chance of having a heart attack. The average for vegan men? Four percent. President Bill Clinton, the guy who used to take reporters to McDonald's *during his morning run,* went vegan after his last massive heart attack. Hardly a week goes by that doesn't see the release of a new study extolling the health benefits of eating plant-based foods. Of the top ten leading causes of death in the United States, stuffing your face with animal-free foods can cut down your chances of developing four of them (those would be heart disease, cancer, stroke, and diabetes, according to the Centers for Disease Control). Every system in the body is bettered by an influx of fresh, wholesome nutrients, which are easily and abundantly found in plants.

THE ENVIRONMENT

The ways in which switching to a plant-based diet benefit our blue-green marble are a matter of simple efficiency. It goes something like this.

VEGAN PERSON: Plants grow. Vegan eats plants. The end.

NONVEGAN PERSON: Plants grow and are fed to animals, which require a significant amount of land and water to live. The animals convert the plants into muscle and are then sent to slaughter. A person eats parts of the animal, getting only a fraction of the original energy input that he or she could have easily gotten from eating the plants directly. The equation simply doesn't balance out, considering how much more

LOVE THE EARTH? DO THE MATH.

It takes more land and water to make food for people when they are eating meat.

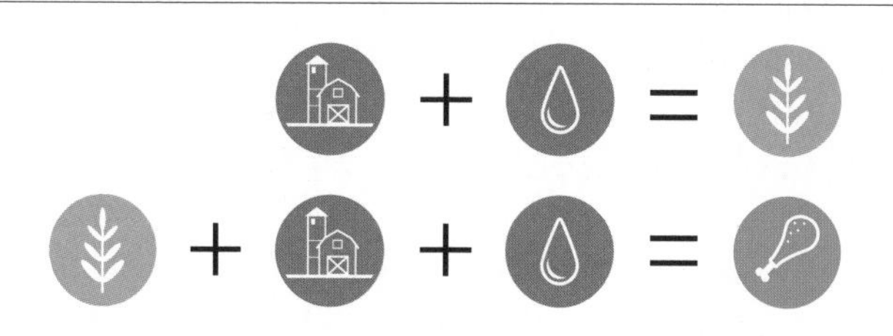

KEY: = water = land = plants = meat

input it takes to yield the same amount of food when the plants are first fed to an animal and then to humans.

Why bother with the middleman (aka the animals that are converting the plants into only a sliver of the nutrients you'd get from eating the plants themselves), especially considering the land, water, and effort required to grow the plants that become animal feed? Each additional step in this process reduces the efficiency of food production, costing valuable resources that could otherwise be used to grow a greater variety of plant foods or using the grains we already grow to feed people directly. Plus, there are the issues of monocrop culture (growing the same crop year after year on the same land without rotation, which damages the soil, the crop, and more) and genetically modified organisms. GMOs are plants or animals with engineered DNA—think Frankenstein, but for the food we eat! Both soy and corn, two of the main crops grown for animal feed, are almost completely GMO in the United States.

Also, on factory farms there are such things as manure lagoons, which routinely leak into and contaminate nearby waterways with their effluent (a much more dignified term for what could easily be called "poop soup"), not to mention their lovely habit of polluting the surrounding air with particulate fecal matter. Particulate. Fecal. Matter. (PFM.) We can probably all agree that decreasing the amount of PFM in the world is a good thing.

ANIMALS

You know how people spend literally billions of dollars per year on dog food, dog clothes, dog tags, dog toys, and other dog accoutrements? It's legit; dogs are adorable. But here's a little logic problem. Imagine the world's ultimate dog: the nicest, most loyal, cutest, and best overall dog that has ever been. This dog lets you take photos of his embarrassing moments, cuddles you when you're sick, and spins around after his tail in little dog circles whenever he remembers that he has a tail. Now imagine that through no fault of his own, this phenomenal creature gets

"We can see quite plainly that our present civilization is built on the exploitation of animals, just as past civilizations were built on the exploitation of slaves, and we believe the spiritual destiny of man is such that in time he will view with abhorrence the idea that men once fed on the products of animals' bodies."

—DONALD WATSON,
in the first issue of *The Vegan News,* his newsletter

Meet This Vegan: BILL CLINTON

That's right: the sax-playing former president is the poster boy for going 90 percent vegan (he cops to eating an occasional piece of fish) after switching to a plant-based diet in 2010. Following a quadruple-bypass surgery in 2004 and another open-heart procedure in 2010, President Clinton began to completely revamp his erstwhile burgercentric diet under the advisement of Dr. Dean Ornish and Dr. Caldwell Esselstyn. In a 2011 interview on CNN with Dr. Sanjay Gupta, Clinton revealed that he sees his former eating habits as "playing Russian roulette" with his health, needlessly risking further procedures and the very real threat of a major heart attack. Now that he's nearly back to the weight he was in high school, Clinton's vitality is as evident as his satisfaction with a plant-based diet.

thrust into a hot dog costume, one of those horribly awkward, totally humiliating whole-body deals that completely masks his incredible nature and turns him into a fast-food stand-in. It's still the same guy inside, but now he looks like a hot dog. This is essentially what happens to the more than 10 billion animals killed for food in the United States every year. Inside the steak, hot dog, nugget, and burger costumes that society forces them into, the cows, pigs, chickens, and other animals we raise for food have many of the same basic characteristics as our beloved dogs. They have brains, spinal cords, pain receptors, personalities, memories, and emotions. They are scared as they stand in line at the slaughterhouse. (For anyone who has a hand raised right now and wants to cry "anthropomorphism"—first, nice vocabulary! Second, consider the fact that autistic animal scientist and author Temple Grandin, who feels a particularly strong connection with animals, has made an entire career, often bankrolled by meat producers, of mitigating animals' emotions as they are on their way to the killing floor.) Animals—including the ones we kill for food—have rich emotional lives: they are happy when with their friends; they mourn their dead; and they protect their babies. If the idea of a dog going through a slaughterhouse makes you cringe, consider taking other animals out of their costumes.

OTHER PEOPLE

Sadly, the lives of today's slaughterhouse workers are just as rife with horror—in many cases, much more so!—as when Upton Sinclair penned *The Jungle* in 1906. They have some of the highest on-the-job injury rates of any profession, both physically and psychologically. A major factor for many people who adopt plant-based diets is the desire to decrease suffering, including that of other humans.

Meet This Vegan: WOODY HARRELSON

Whether he's fighting zombies or a natural born killer, Woody Harrelson's personal life is somewhat more peaceful than his fictional one on the screen—the actor is a longtime vegan. While filming *Zombieland*, in which his character is obsessed with Twinkies, Harrelson had vegan versions made. A passionate environmentalist, he adopted the diet while trying to impress a girl. When he was in his early twenties, a young lady suggested to him that if he ditched dairy, his skin would clear up, and the rest is history. Harrelson was named the Sexiest Vegetarian of 2012 by PETA.

THE PROS

There are a few organizations that do inspiring and momentous work on behalf of animals. Many of them offer veggie starter kits, handy facts, and current news on animal protection, along with recipes and other resources. For specific questions, and how to become more involved, these groups should be your first stops (see Resources).

The Humane Society of the United States (HSUS)

The country's biggest animal-protection organization, HSUS works on a multitude of campaigns, including farm animal protection, animal fighting and cruelty, puppy mills, and more.

People for the Ethical Treatment of Animals (PETA)

This organization has created some of the most effective advertising campaigns of all time, especially around the issue of fur.

Physicians Committee for Responsible Medicine (PCRM)

Based in Washington, D.C., and dedicated to raising awareness of the health benefits of a plant-based diet, PCRM is a go-to organization for current research, helpful programs, and recipes.

Compassion over Killing (COK)

COK focuses on influencing corporate policies, such as convincing producers of veggie burgers to remove eggs from their recipes, making the products vegan.

Mercy for Animals (MFA)

This powerhouse organization has produced some of the most horrifying undercover investigations of factory farms, which have resulted in legal prosecution and felony convictions for animal cruelty.

A Brief History of Veganism

Plant-based eating has been enjoying a moment in the spotlight in recent years (thanks, President Clinton!), but the ideas behind it are far from passing fancies. The word *vegan* was coined by Donald Watson, a British teacher, who adopted the diet in the 1940s and founded the Vegan Society, a social club that worked together to end animal exploitation. In part, Watson's stance as a pacifist came into play in launching the vegan movement, as he objected to the violence of World War II and sought to rid his life of needless violence, including that done to animals.

But even before Watson gave the world a new word, the idea of eliminating animal products from the diet arose from religious beliefs in cultures around the globe. Many Buddhists, Jains, and Seventh-Day Adventists follow veg diets to achieve various goals, such as lessening their karmic debt or maintaining good health as an expression of gratitude for their lives. In the sixth century, Buddhist monks in Japan created shojin ryori cuisine, a form of completely vegetarian cooking that highlights the simple tastes of fresh ingredients, prepared in a careful, thoughtful process, reflective of Buddhist abstinence principles. The Seventh-Day Adventists who live in Loma Linda, California, have gained national recognition for having the longest life expectancies of any community in the United States due to their lifestyle choices, including vegetarianism.*

* Dan Buettner, *The Blue Zones: Lessons for Living Longer from the People Who've Lived the Longest* (Monterey, Calif.: National Geographic, 2010), 117–62.

A DAY IN THE LIFE OF A VEGAN, THEN AND NOW

	1970	2014
BREAKFAST	Granola and powdered soy milk	Spinach-Tomato Frittata (page 154) and a hazelnut-soy latte
LUNCH	Groats, side of dulse	Chopped salad with chickpeas and avocado, side of vegan "chicken" tenders
DINNER	Celery and loneliness	Three-layer lasagne, kale salad, garlic bread, a glass of Zinfandel

Meet This Vegan: JESSICA CHASTAIN

Not only is basically every single person in Hollywood obsessed with Jessica Chastain, but the redheaded beauty also happens to have another segment of fans: animals. Chastain attributes her lithe figure to veganism—although she also attributed her more buxom form for her role in *The Help* to vegan ice cream and meat-free fried "chicken." While shooting *Zero Dark Thirty*, Chastain and director Kathryn Bigelow shared cute animal videos to keep themselves from being drawn too deeply into their harrowing subject matter.

The Timing

Ideologically there's never a better time than now to do something you've been wanting to do, but historically there's also never been a better time to be vegan. There are now more options for vegans than ever on restaurant menus and grocery store shelves. There are horror stories from vegans in the 1970s who had to use dehydrated soy milk powder to make their morning bowl of cereal. Today, walk into any market and you'll find ten brands of almond-coconut milk blends, and every Starbucks can pour a hazelnut-soy latte (which is delicious, for the record); it's enough for a Bill Cosby–style rambling rant. Even people who aren't—and don't intend to be—vegan consume animal-free products such as nondairy cheese or beefless burgers, usually out of concern for their health or the environment. Hardly a week goes by that doesn't see the opening of another plant-based restaurant or a vegan product launch. Basically, being vegan is a piece of cake. Oh, yes—vegans eat cake.

Pro Tip

Wanna strut your newly vegan stuff? Dig into a luscious vegan cake on November 1, which is World Vegan Day. (And, really, does anyone need an excuse for cake?)

THE STATS

In the United States, roughly 1 percent of the population identifies as vegan, and 47 percent of the population eats vegetarian meals on occasion, according to a study conducted for the Vegetarian Resource Group.*

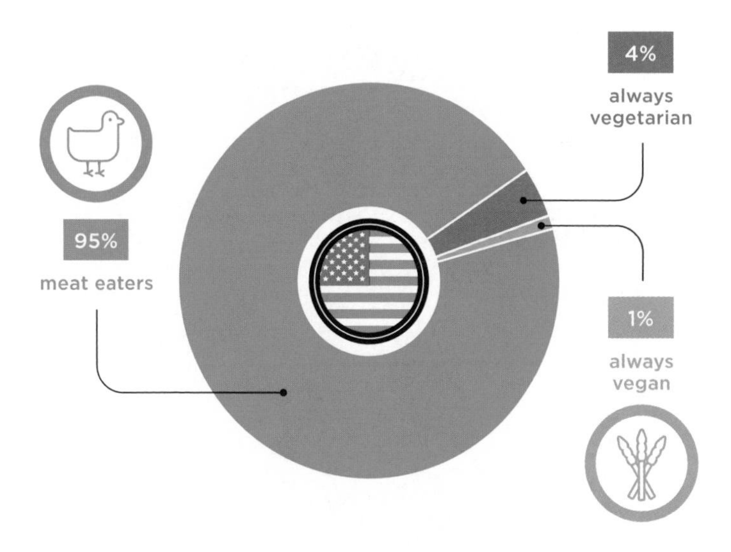

* "How Often Do Americans Eat Vegetarian Meals? And How Many Adults in the U.S. Are Vegetarian?," *The Vegetarian Resource Group* (blog), May 18, 2012, http://www.vrg.org/blog/2012/05/18/how-often-do-americans-eat-vegetarian-meals-and-how-many-adults-in-the-u-s-are-vegetarian.

Do	*The best you can*
Don't	*Freak out*

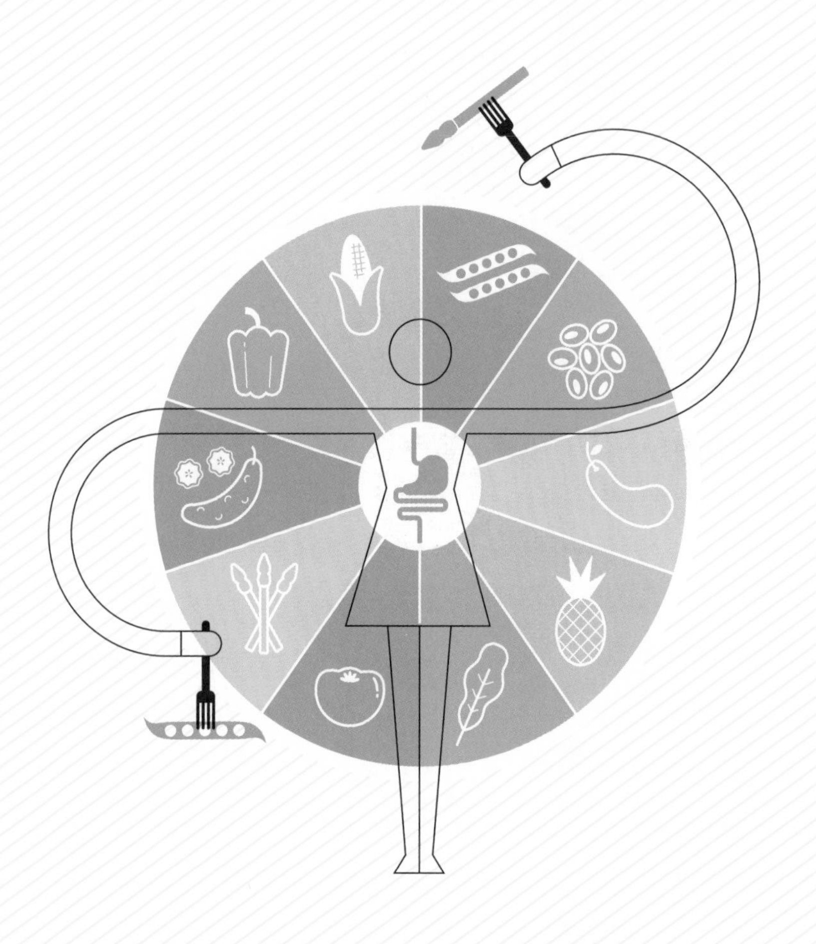

2

THE FOOD

WHAT TO EAT

"People who love to eat are always the best people."

—JULIA CHILD

Is there anything so quintessentially human as the enjoyment of a perfectly cooked meal? We're unique among animals in that we're the only species that sautés, sears, or steams its sustenance. Food is absolutely one of life's greatest joys, for those on a plant-based diet as much as for those who eat animal products. Savoring a perfectly flaky piecrust layered over a rich, homey potpie, biting into a toothsome burger drenched in special sauce, and delighting in the presentation of a multitiered birthday cake are just as thrilling when those dishes are made with plants as when they aren't. Conveniently, eating also gives us energy and nutrients—it's a win-win-win. Going vegan offers a new framework in which you choose what to make for dinner, what to serve at parties, and what to reach for at the grocery store. Cooking and eating on a vegan diet are essentially the same as they are for everyone else; you'll just be using slightly different components. Learning more about new, delicious ingredients, cooking with a variety of colors and textures, and looking at food through another lens create an endlessly fun experiment.

From figuring out exactly how much protein you need and where to get your iron to foraging through new sections of the produce department and deciphering product labels, here's where we get to talk about one of the most infinitely enjoyable subjects on the planet: food.

Nutrition: A Starting Point

First and foremost, yes, as a vegan you do need to worry about your nutrition. But you need to worry about it exactly as much as every other human on the planet—no more, no less. Going vegan does not mean that you'll immediately wither away to nothing or spontaneously combust. Even the American Dietetic Association has stated that a vegan diet can be healthy for people of any age (yes, that includes infants!), and those folks don't tend to mess around when it comes to wackadoo diets.

In 2011, the U.S. Department of Agriculture replaced the long-used food pyramid with My Plate, which recommends making half of every meal fruits and vegetables and the other half whole grains and protein (with more vegetables than fruit and more grains than protein). The switch from pyramid to plate marked a transition for the USDA, since for the first time "protein" did not automatically equate to animal products but instead included plant-based sources of protein such as tofu, lentils, beans, and nuts. The vegan version from the Physicians Committee for Responsible Medicine, called the Power Plate, breaks the recommendations for meals into quarters of a plate, one each for fruits, vegetables, grains, and legumes.

A healthy diet supplies a balance of protein, carbohydrates, and fat (aka macronutrients) and a variety of vitamins and minerals (micronutrients). The amounts of each of these that each person needs depend on age, gender, size, and activity level, so it isn't quite fair to say "all vegans need 40 grams of protein per day" or to give similarly general guidelines. However, you can find out what percentage of these nutrients you need. The U.S. Department of Health and Human Services recommends that adults get 45 to 65 percent of their calories from

PHYSICIANS COMMITTEE FOR RESPONSIBLE MEDICINE'S POWER PLATE

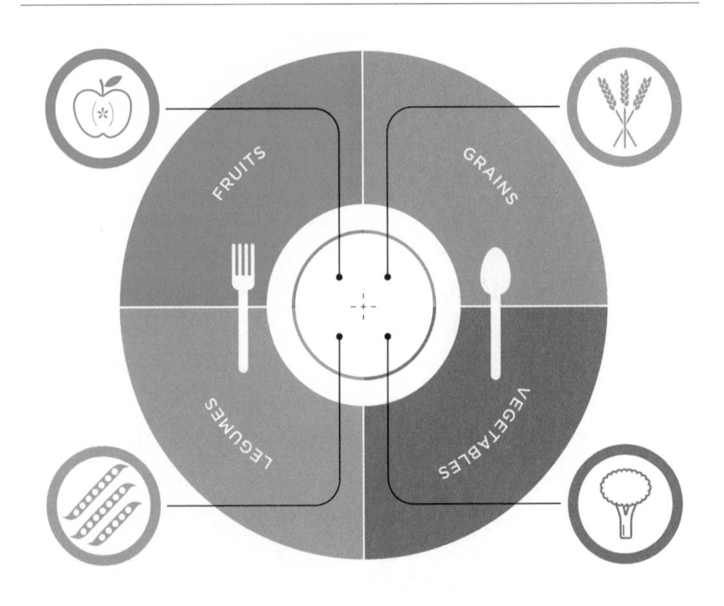

carbohydrates, 10 to 35 percent from proteins, and 20 to 35 percent from fats.* Does this mean that half of every meal should be pasta? As much of a dream come true as that might be, the answer is no. Every food contains a balance of protein, carbohydrate, and fat, so it's a matter of balancing the foods you eat in total. The easiest thing to do is to eat a variety of foods and keep about half of your plate covered in vegetables.

* Percentages from Dietary Guidelines for Americans, 2010, http://www.health.gov/dietaryguidelines/2010.asp.

KNOW-IT-ALLS

When it comes to nutrition, check with a professional. The following are extremely helpful resources.

***Becoming Vegan*, by Brenda Davis and Vesanto Melina**
Written by two nutritionists, this book is the go-to resource for planning out a healthy vegan diet. Davis and Melina plumb the depths of every possible combination of factors—including age, gender, body type, and more—in calculating what kind of nutrients anyone who wants to go vegan will need to stay healthy.

Physicians Committee for Responsible Medicine
PCRM not only offers in-depth nutritional FAQs for both vegan and vegetarian diets but is a leader in current nutritional research. The group also works to educate health professionals about the health benefits of plant-based diets, bettering school lunches, and healing common medical conditions such as cancer and diabetes through diet.

NutritionData.Self.com
If you're wondering about the nutrient breakdown of a certain food (including many packaged foods), check this handy site. You'll find out the food's macronutrient ratio, plus amounts of micronutrients.

The Questions

It turns out that most people really don't know all that much when it comes to nutrition, and telling them that you've gone vegan can set off their alarms. The following are questions that many new vegans find themselves asking and subsequently find themselves being asked by concerned family and friends. Get really comfortable with the responses to these interrogatories—you'll be using them frequently!

Q: Where do you get your protein?

A: From plants. Protein deficiency is essentially unheard of among people who are consuming enough food to meet their daily calorie needs.

Q: What about omegas and iron?

A: You guessed it: you can easily get these from plants as well. Spinach is a powerhouse iron provider; omegas are easily found in flax and other seeds.

Q: Okay, here's a really hard one. What about calcium?

A: Not to be a broken record, but calcium is also available in plants. Despite the very clever marketing job that the National Dairy Council has done (you know, the one with the mustachioed celebrities and poor grammar), dairy actually drains calcium from your bones as it is digested. It would be amusingly ironic if it weren't for the more than 35 million women in the United States suffering from osteopenia and osteoporosis. Leafy greens are packed with calcium, as are sesame seeds and tofu.

Numbers to Know

Here are just a few of the many, many plant-based sources of the nutrients that come up most commonly in conversations about vegan nutrition.* Of course, remember that variety is key. Just because something is at the top of one of these lists doesn't mean you should rely on it exclusively. Vary your vittles!

TOP FIVE PLANT-BASED SOURCES OF PROTEIN

Wheat gluten .... 21 grams per 1-ounce serving

Spirulina (a dried seaweed) .... 16 grams per 1-ounce serving

Soybeans .... 10 grams per 1-ounce serving

Pumpkin seeds .... 9 grams per 1-ounce serving

Peanuts .... 8 grams per 1-ounce serving

TOP FIVE PLANT-BASED SOURCES OF CALCIUM

Tofu .... 683 milligrams per 100-gram serving

Tahini .... 426 milligrams per 100-gram serving

Almond butter .... 270 milligrams per 100-gram serving

Flaxseeds .... 255 milligrams per 100-gram serving

White beans .... 240 milligrams per 100-gram serving

TOP FIVE PLANT-BASED SOURCES OF IRON

Soybeans .... 16 milligrams per 100-gram serving

Pumpkin seeds .... 15 milligrams per 100-gram serving

Sesame seeds .... 15 milligrams per 100-gram serving

White beans .... 10 milligrams per 100-gram serving

Black beans .... 9 milligrams per 100-gram serving

* All amounts from NutritionData.self.com.

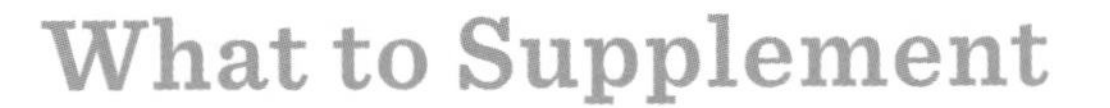

What to Supplement

There is exactly one nutrient that vegans need to take in supplement form: vitamin B_{12}. People who consume animal products get B_{12} from them, and it's not a nutrient that occurs naturally in plants. Without B_{12}, your brain will basically shrivel and die. (No, really: B_{12} deficiency affects the central nervous system, potentially causing severe anemia, confusion, memory loss, weakness, and other horrible things.) It's insanely easy to take one simple supplement, so please do. Yes, many

Meet This Vegan: RUSSELL SIMMONS

If anyone defines the word *mogul*, it's Russell Simmons. The founder of Def Jam Records has helped establish the careers of countless artists. As a devout yogi, Simmons camea to realize his connection with animals after practicing the Jivamukti style of yoga, which was created by passionate vegan activists David Life and Sharon Gannon. Simmons has worked with the Humane Society of the United States to educate the public about the horrors of dogfighting, has been named PETA's Person of the Year, and has also been honored by Mercy for Animals for his efforts.

Do	*Take a B_{12} vitamin and opt for B_{12}-fortified foods whenever possible.*
Don't	*Forget to have your B_{12} level tested during your yearly physical.*

foods are fortified with B_{12}, which is great, but the easiest way to be certain that you're getting enough is to supplement. Doctors recommend everyone take vitamin D, calcium, or iron, but your individual needs will vary—best to check with your doctor.

VITAMINS AND MINERALS YOU CAN GET FROM PLANTS	VITAMINS VEGANS MUST SUPPLEMENT
Vitamin A	B_{12} (Yup. That's it.)
Vitamin C	
Vitamin K	
Vitamin E	
Beta-carotene	
Iron	
Calcium	
Zinc	
Magnesium	
Folate	

Pro Tip

If you're concerned about getting sufficient nutrients, get spicy. Dried spices and herbs (thyme, oregano, dill, curry, cumin, etc.) and chiles are abundant sources of nutrients. It's unlikely that you'll sit down to eat a full cup of dried basil, despite the 2,113 grams of calcium that it would provide, but adding delicious basil to your pasta dish will provide both flavor and nutrition.

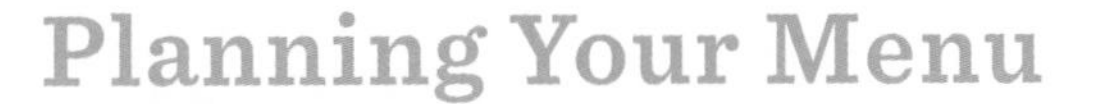

Planning Your Menu

Now we get to the exciting part—thinking about what to eat! Whether you're planning for a single meal or a week's worth of groceries, or just thinking in general about how to approach food, this is where we'll look at what should and shouldn't be in your shopping cart. For recipes, see page 149.

WHAT NOT TO EAT

Let's get the easy part out of the way first. What not to eat: animal products. Meat, dairy, and eggs. Yup, three whole things.

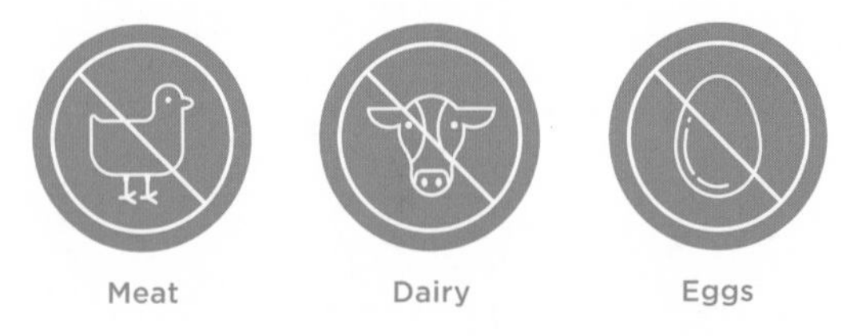

WHAT TO EAT

And now the hard part: choosing from among the multitudinous mouthwatering animal-free options that await. To put it very simply, from here on out, we're eating plants aplenty. But in case what pops into your mind when you think of dining on veggies is chowing down on only alfalfa sprouts and raw rutabagas for the rest of your days, let me stop you right there. Vegans can eat all of these incredible dishes:

- Deep-dish pizza
- Quiche
- Bagels
- Empanadas
- Fettuccine Alfredo
- Double-stacked burgers
- Vietnamese pho
- Lasagne
- Dim sum
- Thai curries
- Sushi
- Enchiladas
- Twice-baked potatoes
- Tiramisu
- Scones
- Birthday cake
- Root beer floats
- Ice cream sandwiches

You get the picture. There are animal-free versions of just about every food on the planet. Is each and every one of them an exact replica of its meat-and-dairy counterpart? Nope. Are many of them significantly more delicious than the cholesterol-clogged option? Indeed! Sure, there are some differences between a vegan frittata and an egg-based one, but, as we all learned in kindergarten, something is not automatically bad simply because it is different.

One thing that most people experience upon going vegan is a newfound appreciation for food. Even if you were ready to riot when the revered food magazine *Gourmet* was shuttered, even if *Zagat* is your sacred text, even if you use the word *artisanal* frequently enough in conversations about food to be a character on *Portlandia*—basically, even if you are really, truly a foodie—even then, discovering the dizzying depth and delectability of plant-based cuisine will curl your toes. There is nothing quite like the thrill of trying out a new restaurant and finding, to your surprise, that it has clearly marked vegan options on the menu. A coffee shop that offers both soy and almond milk? It's enough to make a gal weak in the knees.

PRODUCE PRIMER

It's easy to think that dining sans flesh means you're going to be eating broccoli day and night from here on out. When you actually delve into the diversity of plant foods, it'll soon be clear that eating your way through the produce section is no small feat. One of the easiest ways to make sure you're getting a varied diet is to consume at least three different colors at every meal. Check out these groupings—bonus points for including all the colors in the same day!

REDS: Many red fruits and vegetables are rich in lycopene, among other nutrients, which has been shown to benefit heart health.

Apples	Grapes	Radishes
Beets	Guava	Raspberries
Bell peppers	Onions	Red chard
Cabbage	Passion fruit	Rhubarb
Carrots	Pears	Strawberries
Cherries	Plums	Tomatoes
Cranberries	Potatoes	Watermelon
Dragon fruit		

ORANGES: Feel free to load up on orange fruits and vegetables—there's beta-carotene to be found in all of them, not just carrots, and it's good for your eyesight.

Acorn squash	Clementines	Papaya
Apricots	Kabocha squash	Peaches
Bell peppers	Kumquats	Persimmons
Butternut squash	Mangoes	Pumpkins
Cantaloupe	Nectarines	Sweet potatoes
Carrots	Oranges	Tangerines

YELLOWS: Vitamin C, which is good for your immune system health, is abundant in yellow vegetables and fruits.

Apples	Delicata squash	Pineapple
Bananas	Grapefruit	Plantains
Beets	Lemons	Potatoes
Bell peppers	Onions	Summer squash
Carrots	Pears	Tomatoes
Corn		

GREENS: Chlorophyll—the compound responsible for making greens, well, green—might not sound super appetizing, but it will help keep your circulatory system running smoothly.

- Apples
- Artichokes
- Arugula
- Asparagus
- Avocados
- Basil
- Bell peppers
- Bok choy
- Broccoli
- Broccoli rabe
- Brussels sprouts
- Butter lettuce
- Cabbage
- Celery
- Chard
- Chives
- Cucumbers
- Fennel
- Fiddleheads
- Grapes
- Green beans
- Honeydew
- Iceberg lettuce
- Jalapeños
- Kale
- Kiwifruit
- Kohlrabi
- Leeks
- Lima beans
- Limes
- Oregano
- Pears
- Pistachios
- Plantains
- Poblano chiles
- Pumpkin seeds
- Red leaf lettuce
- Romaine
- Rosemary
- Sage
- Scallions
- Serrano chiles
- Snap peas
- Snow peas
- Soybeans
- Spinach
- Sunflower seeds
- Thyme
- Zucchini

BLUES AND PURPLES: Resveratrol is a powerful antioxidant found in many of these blue and purple foods. So your RDA (recommended daily amount) of it needn't come exclusively from red wine. I mean, it can, but it's not strictly necessary.

Açaí berries	Carrots	Plums
Bell peppers	Concord grapes	Potatoes
Blackberries	Eggplant	Raisins
Black currants	Figs	Taro
Blueberries	Mangosteen	Turnips
Boysenberries	Olives	

WHITES, TANS, AND BROWNS: Paler foods boast their own secret weapon: lignans, which have been shown to reduce the risk of certain kinds of cancer.

Almonds	Garlic	Parsnips
Barley	Ginger	Peanuts
Brazil nuts	Hazelnuts	Pecans
Cashews	Jicama	Pine nuts
Cauliflower	Lentils	Potatoes
Coconuts	Millet	Quinoa
Dates	Mushrooms	Rice
Farro	Oats	Shallots
Flaxseeds	Onions	Walnuts

GOOD GRAINS

Here it is: your first vegan joke. Q: What do vegan zombies eat? A: Graiiiiiiiiiiins. Everyone knows the two most popular grains on the planet, wheat and rice, and their myriad incarnations. But varying the base of your grain dishes is key. Whether you add grains to your favorite soup or blend them into your morning smoothie, they're a great source of fiber. Get to know these less famous options as well.

BARLEY: If you've been consuming most of your barley in its fermented form (aka beer), try it out in your next soup. The plump, chewy grains add great texture.

COUSCOUS: A form of semolina, cooked couscous mixed with any vegetables makes a satisfying meal.

FARRO: A type of wheat, farro offers a shorter grain and a toothsome texture. Great in soups and stews, farro can also make a killer risotto-style porridge.

MILLET: Increasingly popular as an ingredient in ready-made foods like burgers, millet is a small grain that's similar to quinoa in size and texture and offers a light, nonintrusive flavor.

OATS: This breakfast staple will also add a good dose of fiber and protein to your baked goods.

QUINOA: Technically, quinoa is a seed, but most people treat it like they would rice, as a side or a base for stir-fries or vegetables.

LOVELY LEGUMES

Maybe you've never uttered the phrase above. Maybe you should. Legumes are a phenomenal source of protein and satiety for vegans, and to know them is to love them. Like grains, legumes offer fiber, with the added bonus of ample protein. Peas, lentils, and beans are the most common legumes; peanuts fall into this category as well. Think of the warming comfort of a huge pot of lentil soup or the satisfaction of a perfectly seasoned bean burrito—those dishes reflect the best of legumes.

BEANS: Well, I hate to say it, but beans really are a magical food. There are so many varieties that they could fill their own book: black, pinto, pinquito, runner, cranberry, fava, chickpea, kidney, soy, and white navy are just the beginning. Buy them canned or dried with equally pleasing taste.

LENTILS: Whether they're red, yellow, green, or black, lentils are full of fiber and protein. Soups, stews, and cold salads are all amazing with lentils, and you can turn the black beluga variety into a caviar-style dish.

PEANUTS: The most common nut is actually a legume, high in fiber and in protein. Eat as peanut butter or garnish your salads, rice dishes, or even sushi with peanuts.

PEAS: Typically you might not associate peas with protein, but these little green wonders are actually packed with it—in fact, many vegan-meat companies use extracted pea protein as a base for their products.

NUTS, A LOVE STORY

Nuts and veganism literally go together like peanut butter and jelly. But beyond that ubiquitous brown-bag lunch, nuts are nothing short of miraculous. Nuts are packed with calcium, folic acid, magnesium, fiber, and more. Sure, everyone knows (and, by and large, loves) peanut butter, but have you tried the delicacy of almond or pistachio butter? Or almond or hazelnut flour?

ALMONDS: Lightly flavored, almonds make some of the most wonderful nondairy milks, ice creams, and yogurts ever.

CASHEWS: Maybe the sneakiest of the bunch, cashews turn (almost) effortlessly into rich, creamlike sauces in a blender.

PECANS: These dessert stars elevate the richness of everything from pies to oatmeal. Toast them and then grind for the perfect topping on crisps and crumbles.

WALNUTS: Toss a handful of walnuts into your morning smoothie or candy them for a stellar spinach salad. These tree nuts are one of the best sources of vegan omegas.

PROTEIN PARTY

Yes, every plant food contains some of the macronutrient protein, but when you think about replacing animal products in your diet, there are a few items on which you can rely. Some of these vegan "meats" might be new to you, so experiment with abandon when trying them out for the first time.

SEITAN: Yes, it's pronounced the same way that Satan is, but this wheat-based item is more angel than devil. Seitan is the extracted protein from wheat gluten made into strips, chunks, or slices. It's sold on its own and often used as an ingredient, including as the base for many ready-made vegan meats such as sausages.

TEMPEH: Despite its lackluster name, tempeh is downright delicious. This block of fermented soybeans might not sound like much, but when steamed and marinated, it makes a fantastic addition to salads, curries, stir-fries, and sandwiches.

TOFU: Oh, bean curd, where would we be without you? Tofu is another incarnation of fermented soybeans, and it comes in a variety of textures. From the superfirm (best for stir-fries) to the silken (which works wonders in desserts), tofu is an incredible staple.

COW-FREE DAIRY

Back in the day, vegans would make soy milk with a powder that had to be reconstituted with water. These days, the vegan selections in the dairy case are basically spot-on replicas of the cow-derived originals. Milk, yogurt, ice cream, butter, mayonnaise, and cheese are made from almonds, rice, soybeans, coconuts, cashews, oats, hemp, and other ingenious bases. The main challenge is deciding which type you enjoy most.

ALMOND MILK: Lighter than soy milk, almond milk has been having quite a moment over the last few years. There are now truly excellent yogurts, milks, ice creams, and cheeses made from almonds.

COCONUT MILK: In most of the products made with this base, you can taste a bit of residual coconut flavor. Does that make even your breakfast cereal taste like a tropical treat? Yes, but in a very subtle way. There's a richness to coconut milk that's just dreamy in coffee creamers and ice creams. Coconut milk that comes in cartons like dairy milk is lighter than the canned versions. The carton kind is better for cereal and smoothies, while the canned kind is better for curries, sauces, and soups.

SOY MILK: Perhaps the most ubiquitous of the nondairy milks, soy milk is as common these days as dairy, which is wonderful. It's a favorite among product makers for its high fat content and richness. There is a light soy taste (think unsalted edamame, not soy sauce) to some products made with soy milk.

STOCKING YOUR PANTRY: SPEND VERSUS SPLURGE

A common argument against plant-based eating is that it is prohibitively expensive. But, as our old friend logic would point out, anything can be prohibitively expensive if you spend too much money on it. Sure, if you eat the finest macadamia nut cheeses by the metric tonne, gorge constantly on meals at fancy restaurants, ply yourself with costly

Do	*Try out vegan meats and cheeses when you want variety or are craving a familiar flavor or texture.*
Don't	*Think that every single meal must include one or both.*

CHEESE, PLEASE

Nondairy cheeses have experienced a renaissance in the last five years. Here are a few of the most impressive brands to help you begin your explorations.

Daiya Foods

From cream cheese to shreds, this company is largely credited with revolutionizing vegan cheese, because its shreds melt and stretch in a similar fashion to dairy cheese. Pizza parlors all over the country use this brand for their vegan pies.

Follow Your Heart

Blocks of mozzarella, Cheddar, and Jack, plus excellent shredded versions, are available under the Vegan Gourmet line from this dairy-free standard.

Kite Hill

From fresh soft cheeses to aged varieties with actual rinds, this upscale brand offers cheeses that are nut based and treated with the precision of artisan cheeses.

Punk Rawk Labs

Made from macadamia nuts and cashews, these aged cheeses are rich and decadent. The herbed and smoked varieties are jaw-droppingly delicious!

supplements, and wash it all down with Dom Pérignon, it's going to cost you. But in fact, getting the most out of your groceries is surprisingly easy once you master a few simple tricks.

BEFRIEND THE BULK SECTION

Shop around town until you find a grocer with an incredible bulk selection. Go there for all your big restocking-the-pantry grocery trips. Buying staples (think rice, pasta, nuts, spices, snacks, cereal, peanut butter, and, perhaps most important, chocolate) in package-free form cuts down on costs and saves the environment at the same time. A twofer is budget-friendly by definition, right?

PLAN BEFORE YOU PURCHASE

Any human who walks into a grocery store as her stomach rumbles with the first twinges of hunger and thinks, "Oh, I'll just run in and grab whatever looks good for dinner" is a person who is about to spend $85 for the makings of half a dinner, three-sevenths of a lunch, and more snacks than any one person needs in a week, only to realize back home that she doesn't have the can of tomatoes she thought was in the cupboard and her evening meal will end up consisting of toast and defeat. (No, this has definitely not happened to me roughly 800 zillion times. Why do you ask?) Planning out your weekly meals will keep impulse buys at bay and ensure that you're buying things that will actually get eaten, rather than wilt sadly in your crisper. Planning is especially important if you are responsible for feeding others as well as yourself. You might be able to subsist on oatmeal for three days straight, but family members are likely to stage a coup by day two.

SPLURGE WITH SAVVY

Just how critical is it to always buy organic, heirloom, local, artisan, or other adjectives-that-drive-up-prices-but-might-not-actually-enhance-value? The answer varies from foodstuff to foodstuff, but here are some guidelines that will help you make the best choice. Many fresh fruits and vegetables are laden with pesticides, while others are relatively toxin free, even if you buy the conventional option and not the organic; the Environmental Working Group (see Resources) offers a list of the extremes of both, called the Dirty Dozen and the Clean Fifteen (see page 54). For a basic rule of thumb, it's better to go organic for anything that you eat with the skin on (apples, berries, pears, etc.). Items that either come in their own wrappers (such as bananas) or are grown underground (garlic, potatoes) have lower levels of pesticides, even in their conventionally grown forms. Additionally, do you really need the super-fancy pistachio butter for your PB&J? (Hint: no, moneybags, you don't.)

EXPERIENCE ETHNIC MARKETS

Ethnic markets are like Choose Your Own Adventure books: they're full of surprises, they're mysterious the first time through, and once you get the hang of shopping at them, you'll discover new delights every time.

ALTERNATE YOUR ALTERNATES

Vegan meats and cheeses are yummy, they offer variety, and they can ease the path of those new to plant-based eating into the lifestyle. They can also be pricey, especially if they're a big part of your regular diet. Remember that not every meal needs to have a meat replacement at the center of the plate.

FANCY FEAST

Plant-based foods come in all shapes, colors, and, most important, prices. To save or to splurge, that is the question! Make sure to keep your grocery bill in check by splurging occasionally instead of loading your cart with fancy substitutes every time you shop. But even vegans can eat on the cheap. The foods on the left are the best value.

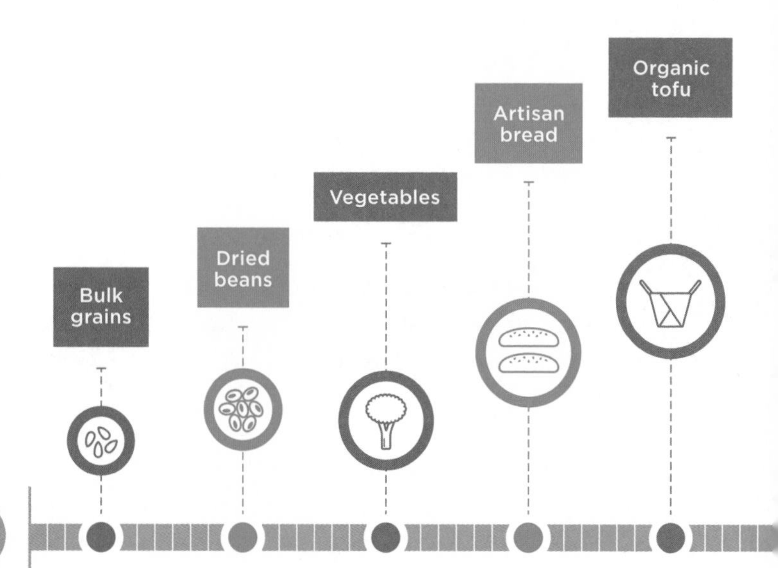

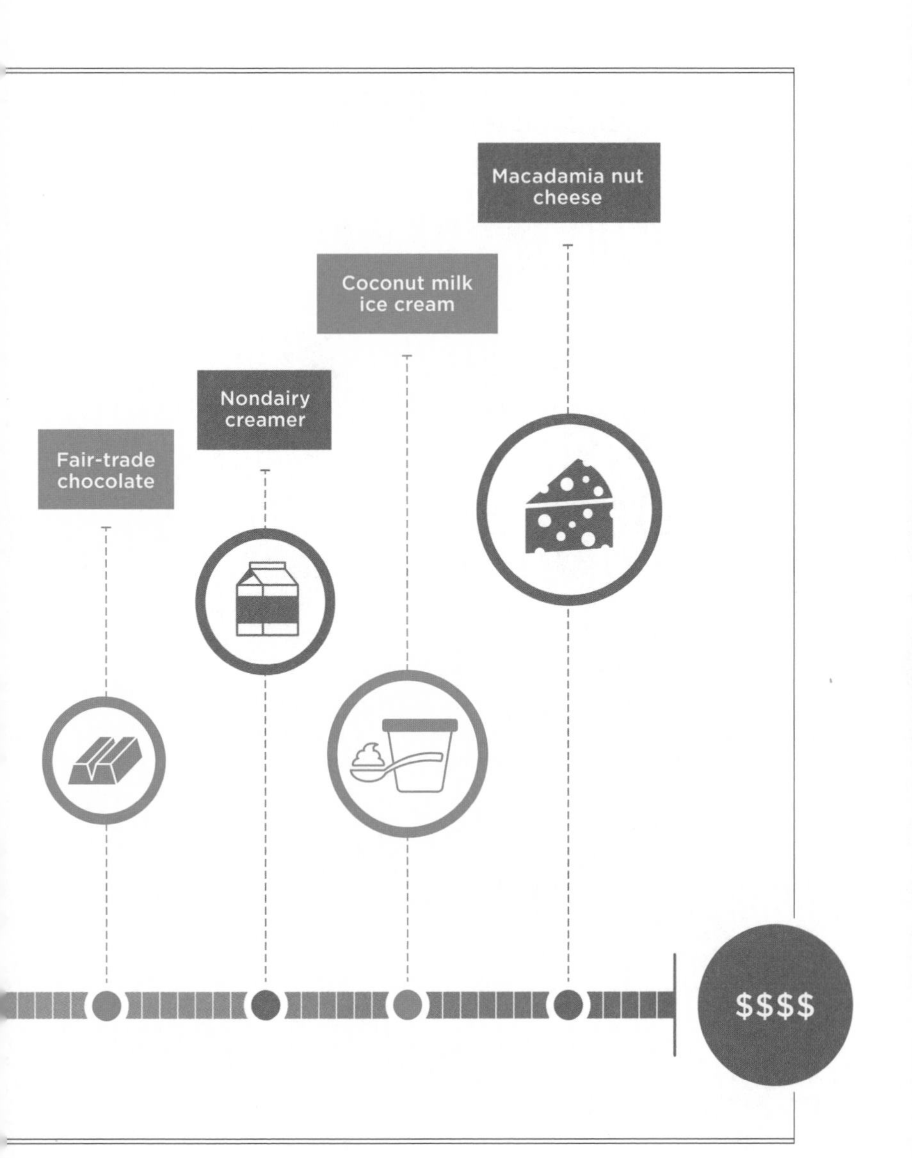
Macadamia nut cheese
Coconut milk ice cream
Nondairy creamer
Fair-trade chocolate
$$$$

WHICH GOODIES TO BUY ORGANIC*

The Clean Fifteen typically have fewer pesticides than the Dirty Dozen. Always buy organic Dirty Dozens when you can, but going conventional for Clean Fifteens is okay.

 DIRTY DOZEN	 CLEAN FIFTEEN
Apples	Asparagus
Celery	Avocados
Cherry tomatoes	Cabbage
Cucumbers	Cantaloupe
Grapes	Eggplant
Hot peppers	Grapefruit
Nectarines (imported)	Kiwifruit
Peaches	Mangos
Potatoes	Mushrooms
Spinach	Onions
Strawberries	Papayas
Sweet bell peppers	Pineapples
	Sweet corn
	Sweet peas (frozen)
	Sweet potatoes

* For more information, visit www.ewg.org.

How to Make Vegan Food at Home

Vegan cooking is just like omnivore cooking. You'll need a cutting board, some pots and pans, spoons—all the regular stuff. Sure, you can throw in fancy blenders and food processors if you'd like, but cooking vegan food doesn't require some sort of secret decoder for cookbooks or high-end kitchen gadgets. Assuming that you already have a basic kitchen setup, it's time to decide what to make. Chapter 6 offers recipes to keep you fed throughout the day. Your next stop? The Internet. There are about a zillion blogs and websites that offer recipes galore. Any specific dish you'd like to make has likely already been veganized by someone clever, and even just poking around different sites is certain to inspire (hello, Pinterest!). But for the times when you have a few things on hand but no clear picture of how to combine them, see the handy guide on page 57. Pick one thing from each column, and voilà, you have a meal. (Okay, fine. You can have more than one veggie per meal. They're that good for you.)

Dizzied by the selection? Here are a few combos that work really well:

- Pizza dough + pesto + sautéed spinach + vegan "chicken" + olives
- Rice noodles + broccoli + tempeh + miso-ginger + hot sauce
- Farro + squash + peas + white beans + tahini + caramelized onions
- Tortillas + bell peppers + black beans + avocado + hot sauce
- Broth + curry + vegan "chicken" + broccoli + scallions + mushrooms

POP QUIZ!

Let's play a little game called "Food or Not Food?" In each row, which of the two things is food on a vegan diet?

A	B
A delicious triple-decker veggie burger with onion rings, avocado, melty "cheese," mustard, ketchup, pickles, tomato, and onion	A cow
A hearty serving of spaghetti and soy meatballs, slice upon slice of super-"buttery" garlic bread, and a salad of greens, figs, and crisp balsamic dressing	A sheep
A huge burrito filled with savory beans, seasoned rice, guacamole, roasted-tomato salsa, roasted plantains, and fresh lettuce	A chicken

Answers: This might come as a shock, but column A has all the right answers. Yes, all of these dishes are available in incredibly good vegan incarnations (see The Recipes, page 149). Once you've flipped through a few vegan cookbooks and spent maybe a bit too much time looking at recipes on the Internet, it will become clear that vegan versions of whatever dish you desire can be made. And the more you experience and enjoy plant-based cuisine, the more outlandish eating animals will seem. If you're perfectly happy with Soyrizo, why bother killing a living creature for chorizo? The inherent violence of eating animal products becomes less and less palatable when you realize that there's no need for it.

A LITTLE FROM COLUMN A . . .

You can make a complete meal by choosing one ingredient from each column. Mix and match to please your taste buds.

BASE	VEGGIES	PROTEIN	SAUCE	EXTRAS
Greens	Root vegetables	Chickpeas	Pesto	Hot sauce
Pizza dough	Tomatoes	Tofu	Marinara	Avocado
Pasta	Fennel	Tempeh	Tahini	Chopped herbs
Rice	Cauliflower	Black beans	Peanut	Sunflower seeds
Rice noodles	Broccoli	Refried beans	Miso-ginger	Olives
Lentils	Peas	Vegan "beef"	Alfredo	Pickles
Farro or barley	Sautéed spinach	Mushrooms	Romesco	Chopped nuts
Couscous	Bell peppers	White beans	Hoisin-soy	Scallions
Tortillas	Squash	Vegan "chicken"	Curry	Caramelized onions
Broth	Artichokes	Soyrizo	Hollandaise	Hemp seeds

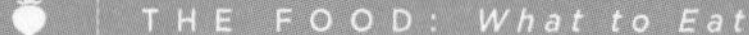

SHOP, DON'T DROP

Although any week's grocery list should be based on the meals you plan to serve, sometimes planning falls by the wayside. In those cases, this roundup of staples comes to the rescue. These items will keep you sustained!

- Peanut or almond butter
- Bread
- Lentils
- Rice or barley
- Chickpeas
- Pasta
- Canned crushed tomatoes
- Onions
- Jarred roasted bell peppers
- Capers
- Broccoli
- Herbs
- Tofu or tempeh
- Almond or coconut milk
- Frozen fruits and vegetables
- Any other fresh fruits and vegetables that catch your fancy!

Meet This Vegan: CARRIE UNDERWOOD

After being raised on a farm and hearing cows call to their family members who'd been sold off, Carrie Underwood decided to ditch meat. The singer then went vegan and has reveled in the health benefits of the lifestyle. When the legislature in Tennessee approved an ag-gag bill (a law that would criminalize the recording of images on factory farms), Underwood took to Twitter, calling for Governor Bill Haslam to veto the bill.

TOP ETHNIC GROCERY STORE FINDS

When exploring your local ethnic markets, make a beeline for these unique, flavorful products.

CHINESE

Although you might never perfect truly authentic hot-and-sour soup at home, Chinese markets are convenience-food-filled wonderlands.

1. **Wonton wrappers.** Oh yes, you absolutely can make cheater ravioli (as well as adultery-free dumplings) using wonton wrappers, which are made of flour and oil.
2. **Vegan meats.** Many Chinese groceries offer Taiwanese vegan meats, which come in flavors not usually found at mainstream supermarkets. Craving vegan shrimp, ham, or fish balls? No problem.
3. **Frozen bao.** Rice flour wraps around vegetables, vegan meats, and red beans in these delectable buns.

INDIAN

Spices galore are what Indian stores are best known for, but they also offer a few surprising treats.

1. **Kala namak.** Also known as black salt (though in color this salt is actually pink), kala namak is key to adding an umami flavor to egg-like dishes such as tofu scrambles and omelets.
2. **Packaged sauces.** If you're craving authentic aloo gobi but not looking to go out, Indian markets offer a bevy of ready-made sauces to which you can add whatever vegetables or other ingredients you have on hand.

3. **Snacks.** From lentil chips to flavorful Bhuja mixes, there are salty, tangy, and sometimes spicy snacks of all shapes and sizes for those who love something crunchy to munch on between meals.

JAPANESE

Far beyond the abundant varieties of rice and ready-made sushi, Japanese markets offer phenomenal sweets and condiments.

1. **Nagaimo.** This root vegetable turns into an eggy miracle when grated and makes amazing okonomiyaki, which is what would happen if pizza and frittata had a Japanese baby.
2. **Furikake.** A condiment made of shredded seaweed and sesame seeds, this salty-sweet gem should top all salads, noodle soups, and rice bowls.
3. **Daifuku.** There is no such thing as being able to walk past a refrigerator full of neatly wrapped rice flour buns stuffed with red bean paste and rolled in black sesame seeds.

KOREAN

Barbecued beef might be the first thing that comes to mind when you think of Korean cuisine, but there's so much more to it than that, including many wonderfully vegan goodies.

1. **Rice cakes.** No, these are not the puffy, mouth-drying abominations that your mother ate in the 1970s to maintain her darling figure. These are chewy little ovals of rice-flour magic that instantly transform soups, stir-fries, and salads into toothsome, satisfying meals. I'd eat these at every meal if I could.

2. **Rice blends.** Usually used to make bibimbap (the delectable dish of rice topped with a truckload of sautéed vegetables, pickles, and a spicy sauce), Korean rice blends include multiple rices, other grains, and dried beans. They make amazing bases for grain bowls and soups.
3. **Gochujang.** This Korean chili paste offers a pungent, earthy flavor thanks to the fermented soybeans mixed in with it.

MEXICAN

Beyond offering dried beans, a vegan staple, Mexican markets are an abundant source for these must-get items.

1. **Masa harina.** This corn flour is what makes tamales possible. It, therefore, is magical.
2. **Plantains.** Whether you mash these big, brusque bananas into tostones or sauté them with rum, sugar, and vegan butter, you pretty much can't go wrong.

Meet This Vegan: ERYKAH BADU

Ageless songstress Erykah Badu credits her youthful visage to her vegan diet. Though she's continually reinventing herself as an artist, one aspect of her life that hasn't changed is her dedication to healthy, plant-based eating. An advocate for animals of both human and nonhuman forms, Badu encourages a holistic, mindful lifestyle.

3. **Mexican hot cocoa.** If it were possible to imbibe this treat—basically, it's hot cocoa preblended with cinnamon and sugar—instead of water, I absolutely would.

MIDDLE EASTERN

Pita and hummus are great, but they are just the tip of the Middle-Eastern-cuisine iceberg when it comes to vegan eating.

1. **Za'atar.** This pungent spice blend adds an amazing herbaceous depth of flavor. Use it with olive oil as a dip for bread, or coat vegetables in it before roasting.
2. **Baba ghanoush.** Eggplant and garlic are blended to velvety perfection in this fantastic hummus-alternate.
3. **Halvah.** Made of ground sesame seeds, this sweet treat is a crumbly, wonderful dessert popular throughout the Middle East and North Africa. Some varieties contain egg whites or honey, but you can also find vegan versions.

Pro Tip

Not every food manufacturing company has its own production plant. That's why you'll often see a little note on labels that says something along the lines of "May contain traces of milk, fish, or egg products." It's not that companies don't know what is in their products; it's that they can't guarantee that a modicum of milk won't end up in their finished items when the company that used the production equipment right before them made Milk Duds, and they need to alert consumers with severe allergies about what they're getting. Most vegans will eat products with these statements on the labels since the trace amounts are (a) tiny and (b) not purposefully included.

Surprise, It's Vegan!

Well-intentioned animal lovers aren't the only folks producing vegan food—it's often cheaper for food manufacturers to exclude animal-derived ingredients. There are a number of well-known snacks that just so happen to be vegan—which is either a blessing or a curse, depending on how much you care about that whole "health" thing.

TOP TEN FAVORITE ACCIDENTALLY VEGAN PRODUCTS	
1.	Wheat Thins
2.	Oreos
3.	Cap'n Crunch
4.	Unfrosted Brown Sugar Cinnamon Pop-Tarts
5.	Fritos
6.	Club crackers
7.	Ore-Ida Tater Tots
8.	Duncan Hines Creamy Home-Style Caramel Frosting
9.	Ghirardelli Chocolate Premium Hot Cocoa, Chocolate Hazelnut flavor
10.	Nutter Butters

READING LABELS

Most vegans can take a ten-second look at any product label and know whether or not the item is vegan—it's one of the superpowers we plant eaters develop. Here's a quick look at common ingredients and their animal-derived status. For ingredients that can be derived from plants or animals, the best policy is to either check the product maker's website to seek clarification or call them directly.

HOW TO READ A LABEL

Yay! It's Vegan	Comes from Both Plant and Animal Sources	Not Vegan, Nohow
• Lactic acid • Maltodextrin	• Mono- and diglycerides • Natural flavors • L-cysteine • Stearic acid	• Whey • Casein • Gelatin • Beeswax • Cochineal • Lactose

Drink Up

Of course, great cuisine would be somewhat less exciting without a delicious beverage with which to wash it all down. The perfect appetite-whetting cocktail or glass of masterfully paired wine can take any meal from good to great, and, frankly, alcohol is pretty dang fantastic in its own right. One surprising way in which animal products are used is in the finishing process for some wines and beers. Egg whites and isinglass (an ingredient made from fish) are often used to remove impurities from beer and wine. The egg whites or isinglass is then removed as well, but for some, their use is reason to avoid certain types of alcohol. Calling your favorite brewer directly is a good way to find out whether animal products are used, as is visiting www.barnivore.com. (There are others for whom this is a nonissue; as with all aspects of adopting a plant-based diet, it comes down to personal choice. Revolutions might not be any good without dancing, and I think they'd be similarly stymied without Champagne.)

Let's Go Out!

Dining out is one of life's greatest joys. The food is made by someone who's been trained, people are paid to be nice to you, and you don't even have to do the dishes. Despite its many enchanting qualities, eating at restaurants might seem a tad daunting to someone new to vegan eating. Not to worry: just as with every single other thing in life, the more you do something (in this case, enjoy delicious restaurant food), the better at it you get. First, there are two kinds of places: the intentionally vegan-friendly restaurant and the accidentally vegan-friendly restaurant. That's right: the vast majority of restaurants are happy to cater to vegans, whether you're headed to a steak house or a juice bar. Here are a few game plans for having a lovely experience at your next dinner out.

IF THE RESTAURANT IS VEGAN: WOO-HOO! Bask in the glory of being able to order any- and everything on the menu. If the restaurant is vegetarian (as in everything comes covered in dairy cheese), it's likely that the server will be familiar with veganism and able to suggest either an adjustment to a menu item or something off the menu.

IF THE RESTAURANT HAS CLEARLY MARKED VEGAN OPTIONS ON THE MENU: GREAT. This means that you can easily choose one of the marked items, but it also means that the restaurant gets the idea of veganism, and, if you ask politely, the chef might be willing to make substitutions. Let's say, for instance, that there's a tofu scramble on the brunch menu, but it's the only vegan thing. If there are other egg-based dishes like scrambles or omelets, ask if any of them can be made with tofu instead of eggs. Nine times out of ten, the restaurant will be happy to oblige.

Pro Tip

Pregame. You have the Internet—use it. Find the menu online before heading to a new restaurant to check out the options. If nothing obviously vegan is on offer, it's a good idea to call ahead and ask if the restaurant will be able to make you something off the menu. The handy call-ahead trick serves two purposes. One: you'll give the kitchen time to prepare, and you'll likely be served something more delicious than if the chef needs to cook something for you on the fly. Two: the restaurant will be aware that there's a market for vegan food. If the chef hears enough such requests, the chances are better that vegan options will be added to the menu or already-vegan dishes will be marked as such. Win!

IF THERE ARE DISHES THAT SEEM VEGAN BUT AREN'T MARKED AS SUCH: NO PROBLEM. Nicely ask the server to be sure that the wilted kale salad doesn't come doused in grated Parmesan and then dig in. When in doubt, ask servers what they recommend for vegans. Most restaurants are familiar with this word nowadays, but if you manage to find one that isn't, just ask what the best vegetarian dish is that doesn't come with eggs or dairy. Voilà!

IF EVERY SINGLE ITEM ON THE MENU MENTIONS SOME SORT OF ANIMAL PRODUCT: DON'T SWEAT IT. Unless the menu is made entirely of animal products, with not a single mention of bread or vegetables, you can ask that the kitchen leave the bacon dressing off your salad or toss together a quick pasta with tomatoes and garlic. If these easy substitutions don't seem possible, ask the server if the chef could prepare something vegan for you and then eagerly enjoy whatever he or she whips up.

IF THERE'S NOTHING ON THE MENU, THE KITCHEN REFUSES TO MAKE ANYTHING ELSE, AND EVEN THE WATER IS BURGER-FLAVORED: OH WELL. Sometimes going out for dinner isn't about the food. Sometimes you're there for a work meeting, for a friend who really needs a good catch-up, or for some other reason that precludes you from going somewhere more vegan friendly. Not every meal will be a mind-blowing feat of culinary excellence, and that's just as true for people who eat mostly plants as for people who wrap their birthday cakes in bacon. Maybe you stick to eating a dry piece of bread and call it a night. Next time, you'll know to avoid this particular spot (or eat before you go).

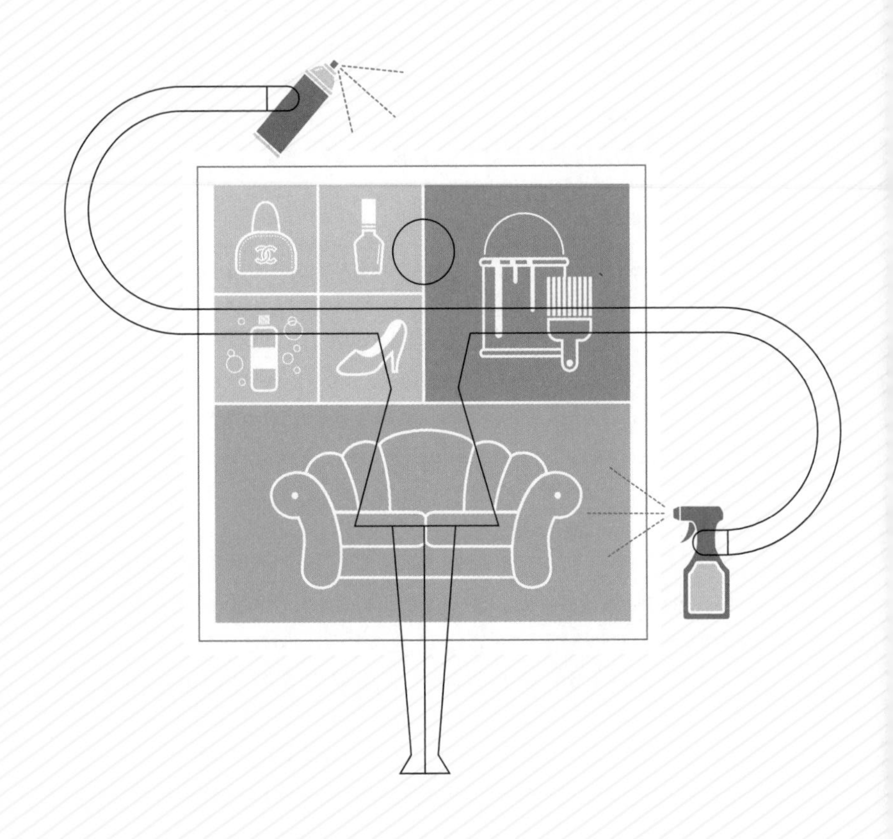

3

VEGAN AT HOME

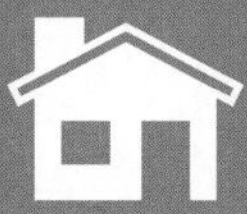

CLEAN LIVIN'

"Have nothing in your house that you do not know to be useful or believe to be beautiful."

—WILLIAM MORRIS

Surprise! This chapter is not about being drug free, although of course it's your house, and if you want to be sober in it, that's your choice. Eating vegan (whether it's all the time or once a month) is a pretty clear concept (yes, plants; no, animals), but what about being vegan in the rest of your life? Cutting animal products from your diet can be a gateway activity to ditching them in other areas, too.

When I first transitioned from being a vegetarian to being vegan, it was partly because I was having a really difficult time justifying using certain animal parts but not others. Becoming more educated about the myriad ways in which animals are (grossly mis)treated for our consumption made me want to spare them at every possible turn. As I mentioned early in the book, living a life completely devoid of animal products is at best impossible and at worst unproductive. But, like many people, I hadn't considered that alligator-skin heels really do come from alligators (having figured "alligator skin" for just a clever marketing ploy, I was shocked to discover the exotic skin trade). This chapter isn't meant to be a banned substances list but an opportunity to consider the origins of some items that might be in your home. Taking a good look at the products you slather on your skin or scrub your tub with can be eye-opening.

First, Fashion

Looking good might be the best revenge, but make sure your retribution reaches its intended target—not a hapless hare. Animals that have made their way into your closet come in forms strident and subtle. Thanks to PETA, everyone and his mother knows that fur comes from the furry bodies of mammals, but wool—so seemingly innocuous in sweaters and socks—is shorn from sheep in a fairly harrowing process. Getting animal products out of the house starts with knowing where to look for them, which animals they come from, and how to replace them.

Does living compassionately mean swearing off designers forever and swathing yourself only in burlap? No! Living stylishly sans animals is easier than ever. From top designers such as Stella McCartney and John Bartlett down to bargain labels (looking at you, Payless Shoe source), there are styles for any taste.

LATER, LEATHER

Leather is really just skin, so if the idea of wearing someone else's skin makes yours crawl, it might be time to consider ditching leather. It lurks in bags, shoes, jackets, and belts, and according to PETA, more than 1 billion animals are slaughtered for their skins every year. One billion beings with brains, pain receptors, and personalities is quite a lot of beings. Whether it looks like shoes or skirts, you can find leather in pretty much every single facet of fashion, which can make it seem hard to avoid. Leather is a by-product of the meat and dairy industries, since farmers can make a profit on cows' skin after their muscles have become meat, their udders have stopped producing milk, and their scraps have been turned into dog food. Cows are by far the animals most commonly used for their skins, but there's also a booming

WHERE LEATHER COMES FROM

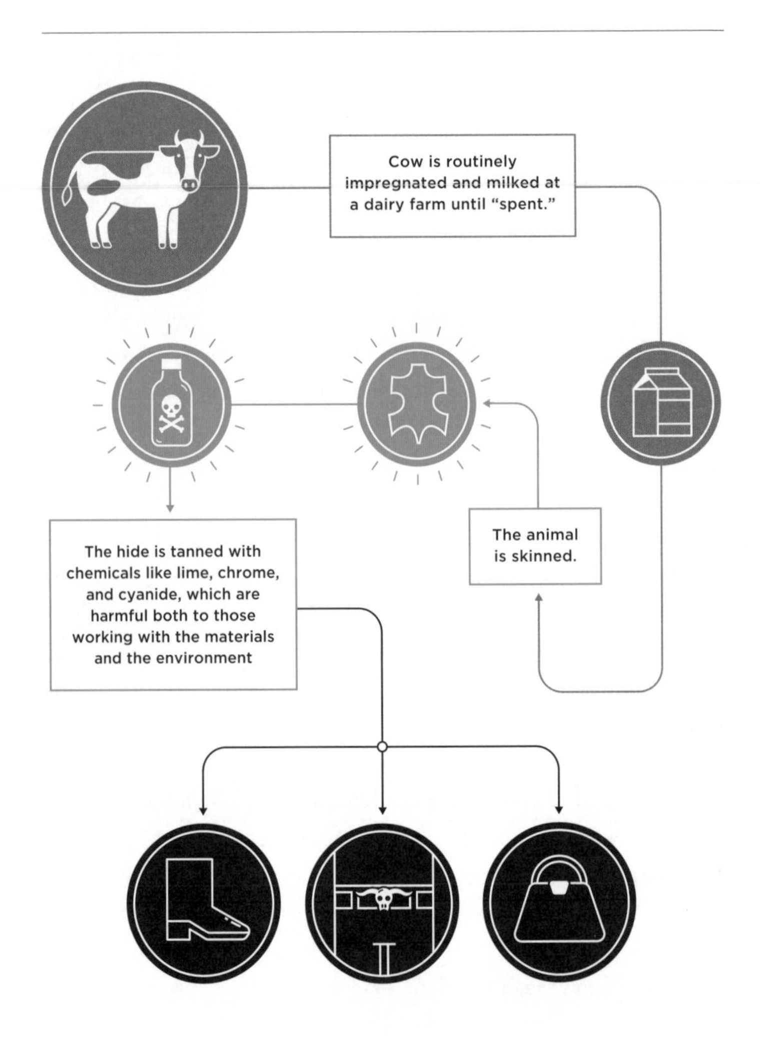

exotic-skin trade. This includes animals such as alligators, ostriches, and snakes that are killed specifically for their skins, though their meat is often also eaten. The exotic skins usually become bags, shoes, and wallets because of their unique appearances.

Producing leather isn't just a matter of hanging the skins out to dry and then sewing them into pants. Tanning is a process that involves using large amounts of chemicals such as formaldehyde, chrome, cyanide, and arsenic, which are not only bad for the environment but also harmful to the people who work with them.

WOOLLY BULLY

Most people think of wool procurement as sheep getting a friendly haircut at the local salon and then returning refreshed to the vast fields of velvety grass, where they roam happily all day long. Unfortunately, the reality of wool production is very different. For sheep—animals so clever that they can recognize *photos* of other individual sheep—being brought up to become wool-producing machines means tail docking (having the ends of their tails snipped off) and castration (for the boys), both procedures that are typically done without any anesthetic. Shearing, like slaughtering, is done for maximum efficiency, so sheep regularly get cut by hasty shearers.

Pro Tip

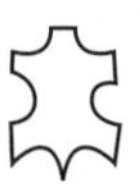

Want an easy way to know whether or not you're sporting leather? Check for the little animal-rug-shaped symbol on your shoes. If it's not there, you're in the clear!

THE BIG GUNN

Thank heavens for Tim Gunn. The *Project Runway* star, *Biggest Loser* fairy godfather of makeovers, and total expert on all things fashion is one of the staunchest antifur advocates in the business. Gunn leverages his heavyweight status to insist that Liz Claiborne, where he's creative director, and *Project Runway* are fur free and has written and spoken extensively about how fashion needs to move past fur. If anyone can make a fur-free future work, it's Gunn!

Merino sheep, which produce merino wool, have naturally folded skin and are bred to increase this quality, since more skin means more area on which to grow wool. This often leaves sheep with excess skin, which can become a breeding ground for flies; there are very few things more disgusting than the idea of being eaten alive by maggots that have infested the folds of your skin, but this very thing happens to sheep. The industry calls it "flystrike." In New Zealand, a country where there are nearly 40 million sheep, 1.5 to 2.5 million are affected by flystrike each year.

FUR IS FRIGHTFUL

There's a reason Cruella De Vil is a villain in Disneydom. If the idea of skinning Dalmatian puppies makes you squirm, so should wearing other animals' fur. There's no pleasant or easy way to put this: skinning animals for their fur is a barbaric process. The disregard for animal welfare is at an all-time high in the production of fur. The

FAUX? DON'T BE SO SURE

Here's some good news: the demand for faux fur has increased over the last decade or so as people have moved away from the cruelties of fur. However, this has also created an oversupply of actual fur, and major retailers including Neiman Marcus, Dillard's, and Barneys have been found selling real fur mislabeled as faux. It's both a blessing and a curse that faux fur is now so close to the real thing that the two are nearly indistinguishable (a blessing because clearly there's no reason to buy animal fur, but a curse because just looking at a garment won't give you any insight as to its origins). To learn more, check out PETA or the Humane Society's Fur-Free Campaign (see Resources).

methods used to kill ferrets, raccoon dogs, sables, rabbits, minks, and chinchillas for their pelts are reprehensible. China is the world's largest exporter of fur, and there are no regulations against animal cruelty for the fur produced there. There are also no restrictions on the kinds of animals that can become fur, and dogs and cats are often killed for their fur, too. Sometimes the animals are gassed—a process that ensures that their last moments are filled with terror—or bludgeoned before they are skinned, but more often they are either vaginally or

Pro Tip

Most vegans avoid silk, as the worms that produce it are often boiled alive to keep the silk threads intact. Thankfully, there are many synthetic alternatives. See more in "What to Wear" (page 77).

anally electrocuted. None of the execution methods is 100 percent foolproof, and animals have been recorded by undercover investigators still alive and struggling to escape as workers begin to remove their skin. It's the stuff of nightmares and should not be acceptable in a decent society.

Meet This Vegan: BIZ STONE

You might not know Biz Stone by name unless you live in Northern California, but you've seen his work. Stone is a co-founder of Twitter and has literally changed the face of communication, news broadcasting, and social interaction with his short-and-(sometimes)-sweet platform. Both he and his wife, Livia, made the switch to a vegan diet after visiting Farm Sanctuary (see Resources) and seeing cows up close and personal, and since then he has become an outspoken advocate for animals.

Do	*Think about what the lives of animals used for clothing are like. Are these the kinds of practices you want to support?*
Don't	*Feel obligated to watch the gruesome videos online of animals being skinned alive. They exist, and some people find them very useful motivational tools for advocating for animals, but they are incredibly disturbing, so use that viewer discretion we've all heard so much about.*

WHAT TO WEAR

If you've ditched all the formerly living items in your closet, what's left? Oh, the soft wonder of cotton, Tencel, bamboo, canvas, and linen, plus the whole world of synthetic fibers—yes, the orange-plaid polyester suit your dad wore to prom was cruelty free (at least to the nonhuman animals).

TOP FIVE SYNTHETIC FIBERS: These words on your garment labels translate to "animal free." From stretchy yoga pants (looking at you, Lycra) to cozy sweater (thanks, acrylic!), these man-made fibers are found in all types of garments.

- Acrylic
- Lycra
- Modal
- Spandex
- Viscose

VEGAN FABRIC OPTIONS

WEAR WITH FLAIR

cotton
spandex
vinyl
Tencel
bamboo
acrylic
linen
viscose
modal
hemp

BUYER BEWARE

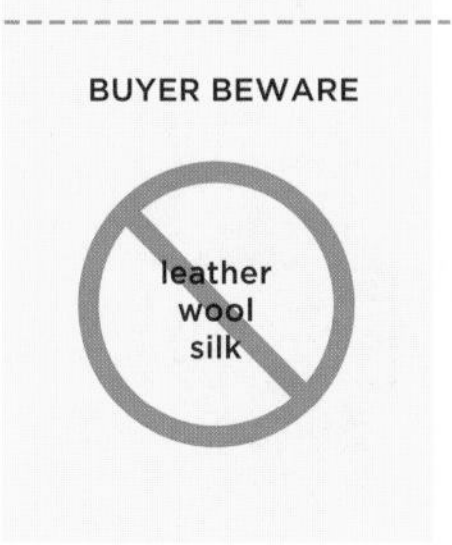

Pro Tip

Try to buy organic cotton whenever possible. Almost all of the cotton grown in the United States is doused with pesticides and other nasty chemicals.

GUESS WHO'S VEGAN?

These days, animal-free duds are nearly indistinguishable from their crueller counterparts. Can you spot the differences between these two dapper gents?

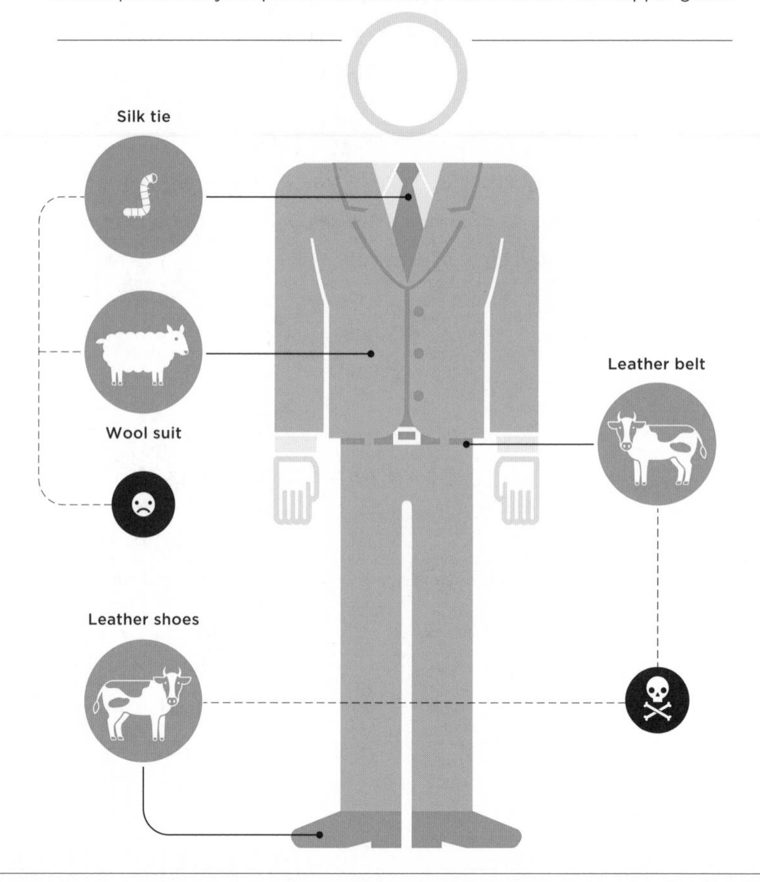

TRADITIONAL MENSWEAR

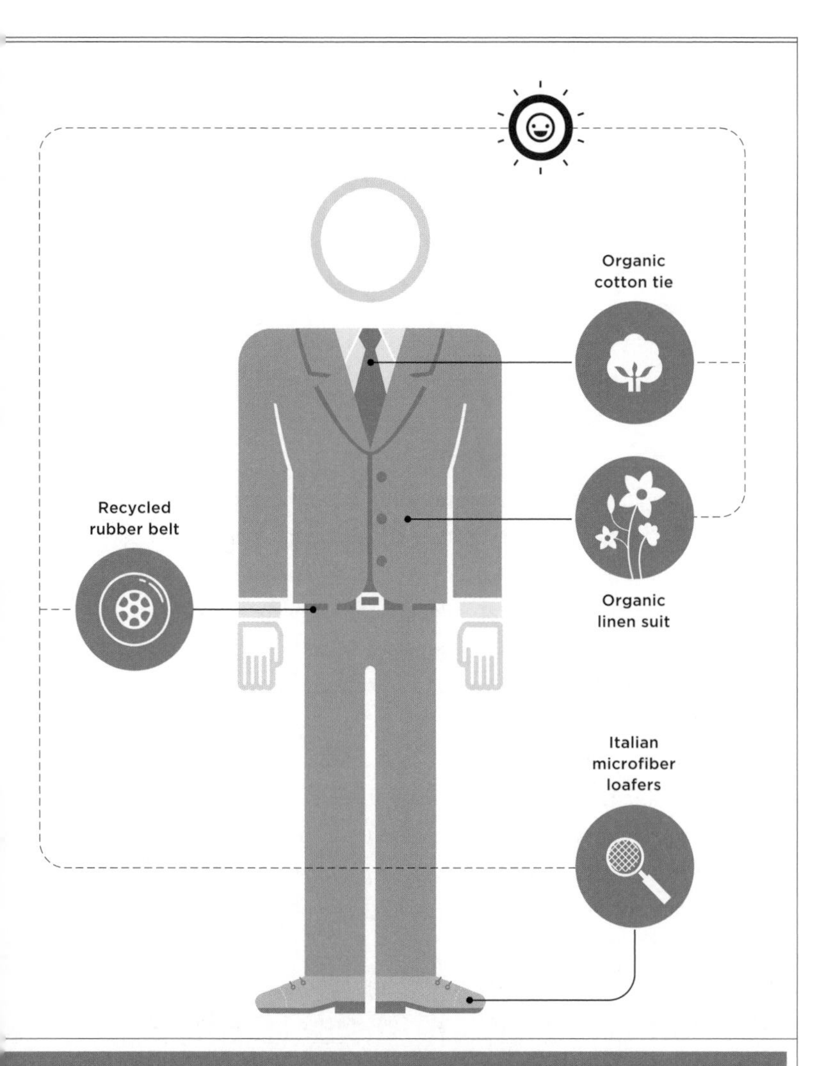

VEGAN ALTERNATIVES

THRIFT SHIFT

Look for animal-friendly wares at these nationwide thrift-shop chains.

- Buffalo Exchange
- Crossroads Trading Co.
- Goodwill

WHERE TO SHOP

So if the idea of sentient creatures suffering the aforementioned horrors turns your stomach faster than a bad matching of prints and stripes, it's probably time to take stock of your closet. Wondering where to buy your threads from here on out? Fear not: there are about a bazillion options. Thankfully, most of the places where you likely already shop have vegan goods aplenty. Here are a few handy lists of sources.

NATIONWIDE STORES: If you're looking for basics, check with the big guys. Macy's, Nordstrom, Bloomingdale's, Dillard's, Kohl's, Sears, and JCPenney are fantastic in that they are department stores, so offering variety is key for them. If the garment tag on something you want to buy doesn't say wool, leather, or silk, it's cruelty-free.

BARGAIN BUYS: The big bargain stores usually offer a great range of vegan items, especially shoes, coats, and accessories. H&M, Forever 21, Target, Payless Shoesource, and Old Navy are good bets for cheaper shoes and clothes.

HIGH-END THREADS: If you're the kind of vegan who hires a personal chef for your daily dinner and frequently jets back and forth to New York just to satisfy your craving for Candle 79 (which would be totally worth it—Candle 79 is a flat-out amazing, completely vegan restaurant in New York City), there are high-end fashion lines just for you! Check out Stella McCartney, John Bartlett, Imposter, Beyond Skin, Love Is Mighty, and Cornelia Guest handbags.

THRIFT SHOPS: If there is any greater joy than finding something that fits you perfectly, is free of animal products, and costs only $10, it's unknown to humankind. Thrift stores and consignment shops are incredible treasure troves of gently used stuff. Shopping at these places is a major boost to the environment—since even animal-free clothes obviously still take a good number of resources to produce—and they are also a wallet-friendly way to restock your closet.

SPECIFICALLY VEGAN LINES: Don't miss the following excellent and purposefully vegan-by-design clothing lines. Whether you're looking for an all-weather coat, a cozy hoodie, or a suit fit for Bond, you're all set. Here are just a few favorites—there are others!

- ***Brave GentleMan:*** Joshua Katcher, a fashion-blogger-turned-designer and an incredible activist, creates extremely luxurious custom-made men's suits as well as a range of men's dress shoes and accessories.
- ***Cri de Coeur:*** This fashion-forward luxury brand produces shoes, handbags, and accessories made of organic cotton, hemp, and even reclaimed wood.

- ***Herbivore Clothing:*** Herbivore is the first name in adorable, wonderfully designed message T-shirts and hoodies. Owned by husband-and-wife team Josh Hooten and Michelle Schwegmann, Herbivore is the place to go when you want to literally wear your values on your sleeve.
- ***Matt & Nat:*** Founder Inder Bedi is a longtime vegan who began this excellent bag and accessories company to broaden the range of high-quality products available to vegans. Matt & Nat offers bags from luggage to tiny totes, all in a variety of colors and styles.
- ***Vaute Couture:*** Started by the brilliant, passionate activist Leanne Mai-ly Hilgart, this line of coats, sweatshirts, tank tops, dresses, and accessories is amazing. Everyone who owns one (including celebs like Alicia Silverstone and Emily Deschanel) is obsessed with the coats, and there is no more perfect sweatshirt.

ONLINE EMPORIUMS: Of course, you can find great vegan gear on Zappos, Amazon, ASOS, ModCloth, and eBay, but if you don't want to have to weed through pages upon pages of leather and wool, check out these totally vegan shopping destinations.

- AlternativeOutfitters.com
- forAnima.com
- MooShoes.com
- VeganEssentials.com

SHOES

Shoes are not only essential for, you know, keeping the broken glass and general filth of the streets from coming into contact with our precious feet, but, man, are they fun. First, let's see what you know about vegan shoes with this handy quiz. Which one of these statements is true?

(A) Going vegan means that all the shoes in your closet immediately turn into Birkenstocks.
(B) Vegans don't need to wear shoes. We just weave our leg hair into mats and pad around on those.
(C) Animal-friendly footwear comes in just about the same sizes, styles, colors, and price points as every single other type of shoe.

You guessed it: C is the correct answer. Really, shopping for shoes is a blissfully simple two-step process: Look for the leather symbol (see page 73). If you see it, buy something else. Done. Good bets for finding leather-free shoes include Toms, Payless, H&M, Forever 21, Target, Macy's, Zappos, and Nordstrom. Also, thrift shops are fantastic sources of shoes.

Don't	*Throw out all the animal-derived stuff you currently own. It's wasteful, and the money's already spent. You can always make sure your next purchase is cruelty free.*
Do	*Consider donating your nonvegan clothes to a local charity or consignment shop if you're not comfortable wearing them anymore.*

BAMBOO

Bamboo is one of the fastest-growing, most versatile, and most eco-friendly plants on the planet. If you're looking for sheets to replace your silk ones, (a) welcome to no longer living in the 1990s, and (b) buy bamboo. As an added bonus, bamboo sheets are hypoallergenic and comfy as can be.

BAMBOO BENEFITS

One plant, bazillions of uses. Here are a few of its many incarnations.

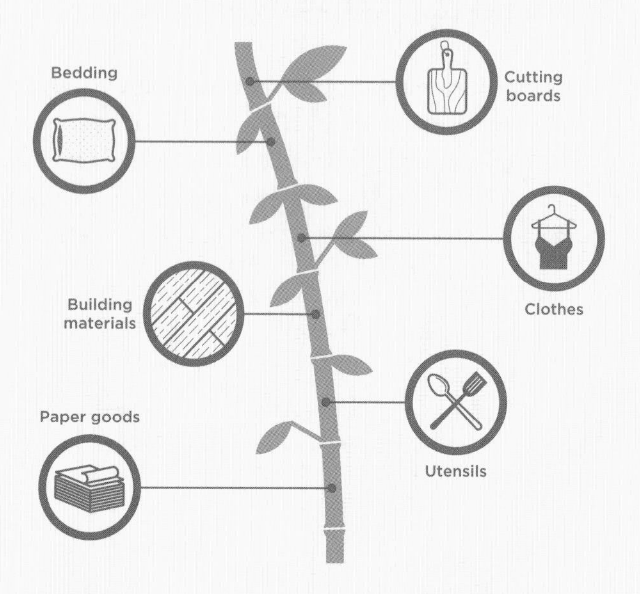

Furnished Fairly

The closet is, of course, just one place in your home. Just as in your wardrobe, leather, animal skins, and fur for decorating your pad are the result of nasty practices, and most vegans kick them to the curb. Leather couches? No, thanks. Sheepskin rugs? Let the sheep keep their hides. Looking through your home to find where animals have become part of the scenery can be an illuminating process. Taking stock of the animal products throughout the house will inform your next trip to Bed Bath & Beyond. (In terms of home furnishings, the animal-free options are usually displayed in stores or listed online right alongside their hide-heavy counterparts, so you don't need to go to Jim's House of Hippie Furniture and come out with a bag full of raffia and woven baskets.) Where you decide to shop for home furnishings really depends on your taste and budget, two things far more limiting than your choice to avoid animal products. The big stores, again, are good bets. Of course, they will also offer animal-based items, but that shouldn't dissuade you from finding just the right stuff for your home.

Don't	*Have a mental break and immediately set fire to all your animal-derived items. That's just wasteful and dangerous.*
Do	*Check out Craigslist when looking to buy or sell furniture. It is the flat-out most efficient way to redecorate, and the environmental friendliness of buying something used gets you extra brownie points.*

THE LIVING (NICELY) ROOM

Turns out that the cowhide rugs that are everywhere on design blogs are just that—cowhide. Ditto goes for bearskin rugs, sheepskin throws, and of course leather couches, chairs, and ottomans. Does this mean you must immediately defenestrate your leather couch? No—think about the passersby! Like all aspects of transitioning to a vegan lifestyle, redecorating to match your ethics (and possibly one of those impossibly aspirational boards on Pinterest) is just that—a transition. Take your time. As with clothing, there's a big market for goods that look just like the animal-based originals, so hunting around for a vegan version isn't terribly difficult.

ANTLER OR ANTI?

There's been an uptick in the use of antlers from deer, moose, and elk in design in recent years. Since these animals shed their antlers as they grow, many artisans create chandeliers and other decorations with found antlers—meaning that no animals were harmed in the process. However, since the antlers of animals that were hunted are also used, it's best to make sure that the ones in your favorite new desk lamp were found. (Side note: found antlers also make great dog chew toys!)

Pro Tip

Yes, the leather couch is an obvious collection of animal parts, but even on fabric sofas, the pillows are often filled with down. Look for "synthetic filler" or "down alternative."

BEDROOM BLISS

This might be the only use of that title that doesn't involve some sort of sex advice—sorry! The bedroom does carry a specific weight when it comes to ethics, though. It's the place where we steal away from the world, wrap ourselves in the most comforting of garments, and recharge. This place has an importance that few others do, and it's essential to feel cozy, relaxed, and calm here. Resting a weary head on the product of cruelty doesn't tend to make for a peaceful night's sleep. The down in your comforter and pillows formerly comforted a goose or a duck, and considering how unpleasant hangnails are, it seems very unlikely that having feathers ripped out is a walk in the park. As we already discussed, wool isn't the result of a sheepish process. As with couches, comforters, pillows, and blankets are available in "down alternative" and in cotton, so look for those.

Bath and Beauty

Although they aren't usually as bold-faced about being animal based as a leather couch is, the products in your bathroom cabinet could do animals just as much harm. The tests that animals endure for cosmetics are mean and nasty. Some examples include the lethal dose test (animals are forced to ingest a substance like shampoo until it kills them to see how much it takes) and dropping household cleaners into rabbits' eyes to measure the amount of damage the cleaning agents cause. Globally, an encouraging trend has emerged in recent years: In the European Union and Israel, testing cosmetics on animals has already been outlawed. Plus, polls consistently show that consumers are against the idea, which helps drive companies to change their methods. Doubt that? In 2008, L'Oréal launched a line of hair care called EverPure, the bottles of which proudly proclaim that the products are 100 percent vegan and not tested on animals. L'Oréal was hardly the first company to offer such products, but it created the line based on consumer demand, and it's added more products to the line since its debut. L'Oréal isn't a completely cruelty-free company, but the addition of EverPure to its lineup is extremely encouraging.

Just as switching to nonleather shoes is not a sentence to wear hemp exclusively for the rest of your life, using products that aren't tested on animals isn't as taxing as it might first appear. Keeping your hair, skin, and teeth looking good without harming animals shouldn't turn you prematurely gray. There are tons of great options—from high-end salon products to drugstore finds. Here are some brands to use as a starting point.

HAIR CARE

Working yourself into a lather should be part of the shampooing process, not part of the process of buying shampoo. Stick with these cruelty-free brands to ensure that your lustrous locks aren't achieved with animal-derived products.

- ABBA
- Adama
- Alba Botanica
- Beauty Without Cruelty
- Giovanni
- John Frieda
- Kiss My Face
- L'Oréal EverPure
- Nature's Gate
- Paul Mitchell
- Peter Lamas

Pro Tip *Dying for a new look? Manic Panic and John Frieda make cruelty-free hair dyes in every imaginable shade.*

FEELING SHEEPISH?

A slew of body lotions—even a few that aren't tested on animals—contain an ingredient called *lanolin*, which is derived from sheep's wool. Keep an eye out for it or look for products that proclaim on the label that they're not tested on animals and contain no animal ingredients.

Meet These Vegans: ELLEN DEGENERES and PORTIA DE ROSSI

Although it's usually rude and unfair to lump a married couple together just because they're legally bound to each other, in the case of this talk show host and actress, it works. The power couple went vegan together after educating themselves about animal suffering and the health benefits of veganism by reading *Skinny Bitch* and watching the documentary *Earthlings*, among other resources. They cemented their dedication to the lifestyle and each other with a vegan wedding ceremony catered by their longtime collaborator, chef Tal Ronnen. DeGeneres devotes an entire page of her website to resources for people interested in ditching meat and often chats up cruelty-free advocates on her show (including one William Jefferson Clinton), and the couple actively supports animal nonprofits such as The Gentle Barn and the Humane Society of the United States (see Resources). As a bonus, DeGeneres is totally the closer for veganism. Whenever people think that vegans are all extreme rebels, a band of unruly, self-righteous tyrants, point to Ellen DeGeneres. She dances. She's funny. Everyone and his grandmother loves her.

BODY CARE

The companies below leave the animal fats (and testing) out of their soaps, deodorants, and lotions.

- Alba Botanica
- Bulldog Natural Skincare
- Crystal Rock
- Dr. Bronner's Soaps
- Herban Cowboy
- Hugo Naturals
- Kiss My Face
- 100% Pure

MAKEUP

Plant-based pigments have been used to adorn the face for eons—some of the first rouges were simply ground plants—but along the way, animal products such as cochineal, a red coloring made from ground beetles, were brought into the cosmetics game. These lines offer excellent dolling-up options, sans bugs.

- Ecco Bella
- E.L.F. Cosmetics
- 100% Pure
- Pacifica
- Tarte Cosmetics*
- Urban Decay*
- Wet 'n Wild
- ZuZu Luxe

*Has great vegan offerings but is not a totally vegan line.

Pro Tip

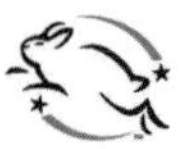

Some products are labeled "Finished product not tested on animals," which means that some of the components of the product might have been tested on animals by whoever developed them (a second party) before they were added to the final product by the company listed on the label. When you're on the prowl for cruelty-free cosmetics, look for the Leaping Bunny. This symbol indicates products that are not tested on animals.

Meet This Vegan: ED BEGLEY JR.

Whether you know Ed Begley Jr. best as the follicly challenged Stan Sitwell from *Arrested Development* or from his having been in what seems like every single TV series ever as some character or other, his most important role has been that of a passionate environmental activist. He's campaigned against the Keystone XL pipeline, is known for riding his bike instead of driving, and is a longtime vegan. Begley is so devoted to the cause of helping the planet that he developed a line of environmentally friendly cleaning products, Begley's Earth Responsible Products.

TOOTHPASTE

If you're hoping to make sure your pearly whites don't come at the cost of animals' lives, check out these cruelty-free options.

- Desert Essence
- Jāsön
- Nature's Gate
- Tom's of Maine

NAIL POLISH

In the last few years, the nail polish trend has absolutely exploded: from nail art blogs to celebrity stylists, nails are now a major force in fashion. Polish up your tips with these bunny-friendly brands.

- LVX
- No Miss
- Obsessive Compulsive Cosmetics
- Rescue Beauty Lounge
- Scotch Naturals
- SpaRitual
- Zoya

Cleaning Products

Cleaning house—both literally and figuratively—can be one of the most rewarding aspects of taking up a new vegan lifestyle. When the purchases you make (whether for food, clothing, or household stuff) reflect the person you want to be, it's so much easier to feel at home.

At this point it probably comes as no shock that the household cleaners that lurk beneath our sinks are often tested on animals, which, of course, is gross. The good news is that thanks to consumer demand for nontoxic products that have not been rubbed into rabbits' eyes, the selection of eco-friendly, cruelty-free cleaners has never been better. Whether you want to go completely au naturel and scrub everything in your home with baking soda and lemon juice or you just need to run down to the corner store and grab some detergent so you can do laundry before having to resort to your absolute least comfortable pair of underpants, you're in luck.

TOP FIVE CRUELTY-FREE CLEANING PRODUCT BRANDS

The following companies offer a twofold benefit: their products aren't tested on animals, and they are significantly better for the environment than the standard chemical cleaners.

- Bon Ami
- Ecover
- Method
- Mrs. Meyer's Clean Day
- Seventh Generation

(PRACTICALLY) PACKAGE-FREE

If wanting to get the products tested on animals out of your house sends you into an eco-friendly fury and you decide to make do without cleaning products that come wrapped in plastic, good for you! Instead of letting your leather-free abode slide into a slimy decline, try using these natural cleansers.

BAKING SODA: Not only do you need this innocuous white powder for perfectly textured chocolate chip cookies, but you can also use it to clean your kitchen. Baking soda is a multitasking wonder: mix it with a bit of water to make a dynamite scrub for sink and counters, leave a box open in your refrigerator to absorb unpleasant odors, or combine it with a small amount of hydrogen peroxide and water to make a (not super-tasty but effective) toothpaste.

LEMON JUICE: There's a reason so many commercial cleaning products are lemon scented: lemons are a great cleanser (and, you know, they smell good, too). You can substitute lemon juice for nearly all of your countertop cleansers. Scrub cutting boards, tiles, sinks, and tubs with fresh lemon juice and then rinse with soapy water.

WHITE VINEGAR: Like baking soda, white vinegar is one of those things you almost always have in the house but sometimes aren't exactly sure why. Well, good news! Drop a cup of it into the sink to destink the drain when needed, or when the drain gets backed up, and let the vinegar work its magic. Use full-strength vinegar to clean your windows and countertops. Mix vinegar with salt to shine chrome sink fixtures. Clean your refrigerator shelves with a solution of half vinegar and half water.

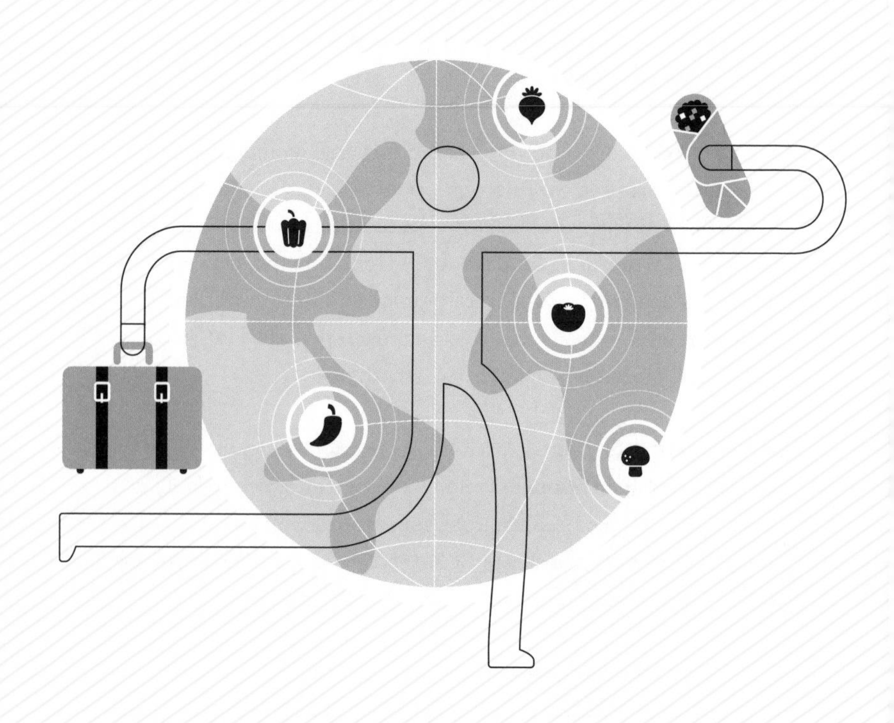

4

TRAVEL

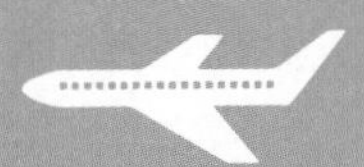

THE WIDE WORLD

"It's a magical world, Hobbes, ol' buddy . . . let's go exploring!"

—CALVIN
(*CALVIN AND HOBBES*)

What's a worldly vegan to do? Get the fudge out of the house! There's this whole huge world, and we might as well take it in, no? Enjoying the exquisite breadth and depth of travel—the foreign streets that feel somehow familiar, the stunning vistas from far-off coasts, the food!—can sometimes be daunting to those who've recently decided to cut out animal products. The good news is that getting around as a vegan, much like traveling in general, is a snap once you know the tricks.

Once they eliminate animal products from their diets, people often discover a whole new world of fruits and vegetables and tend to appreciate them significantly more than they previously did. But there's also literally a whole new world of exciting plant foods that await around the globe. Getting to try out fun new things is one of life's most important bonuses. As Roger Ebert put it, "We are put on this planet only once, and to limit ourselves to the familiar is a crime against our minds." The man had a way with words, but in this particular case, let's change "minds" to "taste buds." From a perfectly crispy southern Indian dosa to an arepa in Venezuela brimming with beans and avocado, there's no shortage of intensely wonderful vegan-friendly food to explore. Oh, and, you know, some sights to see and cultures to appreciate, if you're into that kind of thing.

In the Airport

"All you can eat" takes on a new meaning at airports. Sometimes you'll find yourself staring at a tiny packet of peanut butter and think, "Is this really all I can eat?" When you're new to veganism, it can seem like menus (particularly those at places like airports, where the food doesn't so much come out of kitchens as it does stations and asking for something off the menu isn't always an option) suddenly shrink down to wilted lettuce with salt and pepper. This was definitely much more the case in years past, but airports (especially the big ones) now tend to be a bit more creative-eating friendly. Plus, if you're like me and the thought of flying totally terrifies you, the hunt for something delicious to enjoy can distract you from your impending doom. Total bonus!

GO-TO AIRPORT MEALS

If you're struggling through a long layover or for some unthinkable reason failed to eat before you left home and don't particularly feel like surviving on half a can of ginger ale, you'll need to find sufficient food to get you through your journey. Getting something solid and delicious at an airport can be a tall order (even if you do eat meat and cheese), but there are a few surefire ways to stave off starvation.

1. **A bagel with peanut butter and banana.** These three items might not all come from the same airport deli/restaurant, but they almost always are available. Take the bagel, slather on peanut butter and banana slices, and you have yourself a completely respectable meal.
2. **Soup.** It's not the most exciting thing in the world, but there's something comforting about split pea soup with a nice sourdough roll. My favorite is from the San Francisco Soup Company at SFO

VEGAN-FRIENDLY U.S. AIRPORTS

If you happen to fly into or out of or have a layover at one of these places, good news! Abundant delicious food awaits, before you even get to your actual destination.

John F. Kennedy International Airport

Any major hub is going to have some hidden-gem vegan food, but JFK's gems are right out in the open. Cibo Express Gourmet Market is a smorgasbord of sandwiches, wraps, noodles, juices, and baked goods.

Newark Liberty International Airport

In 2012 the Physicians Committee for Responsible Medicine named Newark the healthiest U.S. airport for food. Shop the Cibo Express market in Terminal B for vegan snacks.

O'Hare International Airport

Do you ever have a layover that isn't in Chicago? O'Hare is an airport at which you can spend an undue amount of time, so finding food is key. This place also boasts Cibo Express markets, and don't miss Burrito Beach—a Mexican restaurant with vegetarian options clearly marked—for something warm and filling.

San Francisco International

Even if you're not flying out of Terminal 2 here, walk over to it and get yourself a burger at the Plant Cafe. This fantastic local mini-chain has a few locations throughout the city and offers travelers salads, juices, and cupcakes in addition to its delicious signature beet burger.

because it's tasty and the company clearly marks the options that are both vegetarian and dairy free.

3. **The condiment sandwich.** Okay, this might not exactly be the most upscale meal of your entire life, but it will certainly subdue the pangs of hunger that only add to any preflight panic. Here's what you do: go to a deli and ask if they have avocado. If they don't, find another deli. Once you've secured avocado, ask for their best roll or bread loaded with every vegetable in sight—lettuce, tomato, onion, the aforementioned avocado, sprouts, cucumber slices, red peppers, peperoncini—as well as vegan condiments like mustard, salt, pepper, and, if they have it, hummus. A five-course tasting menu this is not, but it will keep you from robbing the child in the seat next to you of his Cheerios (which are in fact vegan, in case you fail).
4. **Oatmeal.** When the world is dark and cold (as it often is when you have an ungodly departure time), a nice big serving of oatmeal is the perfect warming comfort food. Starbucks offers a really good bowlful, accompanied by little packets of brown sugar, dried fruit, and chopped nuts. You can also pull the fancy PB&B trick here or get an apple (even the newsstand will have apples), chop it, and toss it in with some cinnamon for a new flavor combination. If you're feeling particularly in need of some comfort, ask the barista to add a touch of cocoa powder or syrup (which they have on hand

Pro Tip

Ask for what you want. The fact that a menu doesn't have all the things you'd like to eat listed together doesn't mean that they can't be served to you together, so long as you're courteous as opposed to demanding.

for mochas), soy milk, and sugar into the mix. If you go this route, offer up front to pay an extra dollar so as not to be a needy jerk. No one likes those.

5. **A burrito.** No, you're not going to find a burrito comparable to those in San Francisco's Mission District (where they are phenomenal, for the record), but you can very likely find a collection of beans, rice, vegetables, and guacamole, and that's no small thing when you're hungry! Not seeing what you want on the menu? If the restaurant offers fajitas, you can usually ask for the vegetables from those wrapped up with rice and beans.

Meet This Vegan: JOAQUIN PHOENIX

Though his enthusiasm for acting has had its ups and downs, one thing that's never wavered in Joaquin Phoenix's life is his commitment to living cruelty free. Veganism was a family affair for the Phoenixes, and Joaquin was raised veg along with his four siblings. During the shooting of *Gladiator*, he requested a leather-free wardrobe for his role as Roman emperor Commodus. Phoenix narrates the seminal animal-rights documentary *Earthlings* and has worked with PETA on many campaigns, including ones that highlight the horrors of the exotic-skin trade and what fish go through when they're pulled out of the water by fishermen.

SHOULD I GET A BURRITO AT THE AIRPORT?

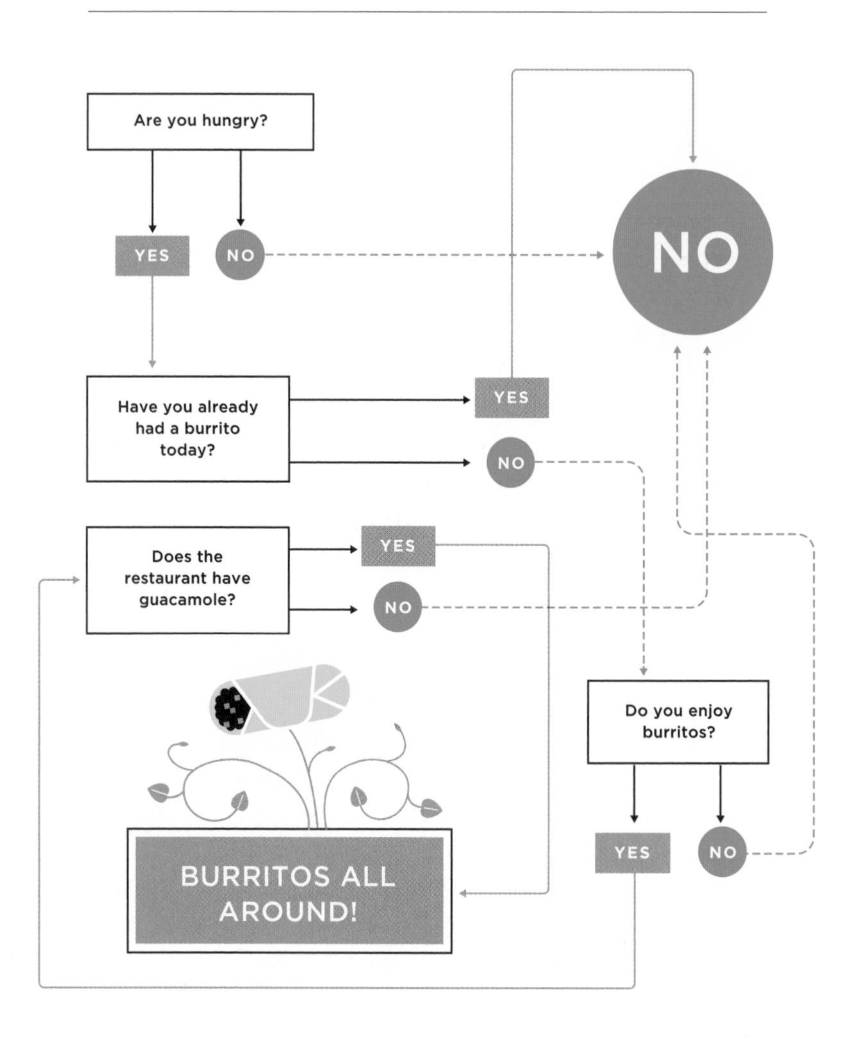

TOP FIVE AIRPORT TREATS

Energy bars, all varieties of nuts, and other overpriced-but-reliable goods are available at airports to ensure that you don't starve to death en route. But beyond the basics, most airports offer a few items that are more like treats and less like basic survival. Here are five vegan airport indulgences.

1. **An enormous (like, to an unwieldy degree) vanilla soy steamer or hot cocoa.** Most coffee shops in airports now carry soy milk, and the warm comfort of a huge, sweet beverage can be much needed during travel. (Side note: for those who do caffeine, an equally huge coffee is also satisfying.)

2. **Sushi.** It's not exactly what you might call cost-effective to buy three trays of airport cucumber rolls in the hopes of totally filling yourself up, but one roll with soy sauce and wasabi can give your mouth a temporary thrill.

3. **Dark chocolate.** One of the best things about airports is that they are filled with items that you're meant to give as gifts to the people you're traveling to see. Sometimes (especially when flying) you might just be in need of an awesome gift for yourself, and dark chocolate fills the bill.

4. **Nutter Butters.** Well, they're just delicious, and vegan, and you can find them in pretty much every Hudson News (the big newsstands in U.S. airports) in the country. Plus, clearly, the most fun thing about being at an airport is perusing the magazine covers, trying

to decide which one to buy, panicking about picking the wrong one, then buying three titles instead of just one and subsequently lugging around a much heavier bag than you had when you left home.

5. **Booze.** Who's kidding whom here? If you're stuck somewhere, getting a drink is a great way to pass the time, make new friends, and enjoy yourself. (Frankly, this is just as true at a co-worker's birthday party as it is at the airport!) Every major airport has a selection of bars, so belly up and quench your thirst.

Meet This Vegan: JOHN SALLEY

Are you ready for the pun to come? Veganism is a slam dunk for former NBA star John Salley. Though he didn't completely ditch animal products until his days on the court were over (in 2007), Salley has been a tireless advocate for healthy living, often saying that had he known in his youth what he does today about the benefits veganism has for physical health, he'd still be playing. Salley has worked with PETA and Physicians Committee for Responsible Medicine and has partnered with a number of fledgling vegan companies.

Pro Tip

There are some restaurants that put dairy in guacamole (sacrilege, I know!), so if the guac in front of you is more the color of Kermit the Frog than avocados, it might be a good idea to double-check that it's dairy free.

On the Ground, Around the World

Before heading out into the world, check and see what the veg-friendly regional dishes of your destination are. (If you're going to Antarctica, best of luck. Pack extra Clif bars.) As always, a quick Internet search is your trusty friend for finding the best of wherever you're headed. Fun fact: even in Ulan Bator, the capital of Mongolia, a country where the traditional diet is yak based, there are eight completely vegan restaurants! As I mentioned in Chapter 2, what we call "ethnic cuisine"—in the countries from which it originates, it's just called "dinner"—can be a smorgasbord of vegan opportunity.

And there's one other little consideration to keep in mind while traveling: it's not always about the food (see Antarctica). Sometimes the trip is about the trip: getting to see a new part of the world, visiting an old friend, experiencing a particular event, or any of the other hundreds of reasons to get off your couch. If you're traveling specifically to eat yummy things, do your research before you go and seek out all the

START HERE

The first step to any trip (whether in the United States or abroad) for a vegan should be to visit the website HappyCow .net, which lists all the vegan, vegetarian, and veg-friendly restaurants in every city in the world, along with health food stores and other local resources. It is an absolute must for planning.

vegan hot spots at your destination. If you're more of the throw-a-dart-at-a-map-and-go-there type of traveler, familiarize yourself with commonly found veg dishes.

AFRICA

Stews, grains, and veggies simmered in pungent spices are the hallmarks of African vegan food.

BERBERE: An Ethiopian spice mix made of garlic, red pepper, and other spices, it's used in rubs, sauces, and condiments to give a kick of heat to many African dishes.

POTATO-PEANUT STEW: A hearty blend of vegetables and peanuts (one of the primary sources of vegan protein in African cuisine), stews like this one are found throughout the continent.

INJERA: This spongy teff-based sourdough bread is the foundation of every Ethiopian platter. The bread soaks up the rich stewed vegetables that sit on top of it and doubles as edible silverware.

WAT: In Ethiopia, wats are the stewed vegetables and lentils that come on top of injera. Collard greens and yellow split peas are popular versions.

JOLLOF RICE: Another transcontinental staple, jollof rice is typically flavored with tomatoes, onions, and spices but can also include vegetables (and meat, so be sure to check on what variety you're getting).

ASIA

Throughout Asia, rice and vegetables are staples, and meat is often used only as a flavoring or topping. Plus, this is the birthplace of tofu, which makes it the default vegan motherland.

BUBBLE TEA (OR BOBA): If you are in Taiwan or Korea, get thee a bubble tea. This luscious drink blends soy milk, an accent flavor, and delightfully chewy tapioca balls together into the perfect cool-down drink. Fun fact: most bubble tea places list "milk" on the menu but offer vegan options such as soy milk since lactose intolerance is so prevalent in Asia.

JAPCHAE: Glass noodles meet slivered vegetables and a savory soy-based sauce in this fantastic Korean dish.

Meet This Vegan: ALICIA SILVERSTONE

It has to be said: when it comes to protecting animals, actress Alicia Silverstone is anything but clueless. A vegan since back in the 1900s (1999, to be exact), she published *The Kind Life*, her first book, in 2009 and followed it up with a community website of the same name. Silverstone never misses an opportunity to help educate about veganism, having appeared on both Oprah's and Ellen DeGeneres's shows to advocate for healthy, eco-friendly living. Her next projects include two more Kind books, one about parenting and a cookbook.

SPRING ROLLS: Whether you're in Thailand or Vietnam, there's nothing like a selection of fresh vegetables and herbs wrapped in chewy, perfect rice paper and dipped into a savory sauce.

SHOJIN RYORI: This isn't a dish but a style of Japanese cuisine that focuses on lengthy and intricate cooking techniques for vegetables. Look for a monastery that offers meals in this style.

BIBIMBAP: A Korean stunner in which a blend of rices is mixed with steamed, sautéed, and pickled vegetables and tossed together with a rice wine sauce.

EASTERN EUROPE

Of course, there's no shortage of good vodka to be found once you get east of Austria, but you might be surprised to find that there's some highly hearty animal-free food to enjoy in between drinks.

BORSCHT: A gorgeous crimson soup made of fresh beets and garnished with dill, borscht is a traditional Russian dish. Make sure to leave off the dollop of sour cream that usually accompanies it.

PIEROGIS: As with all the world's delicious dumplings, these delightful doughy pockets can be filled with anything; potatoes are a common stuffing.

CABBAGE ROLLS: These savory treats might not have the most glamorous name ever, but they'll satisfy. Steamed cabbage is rolled around rice and stewed in tomato sauce for a nice, light meal.

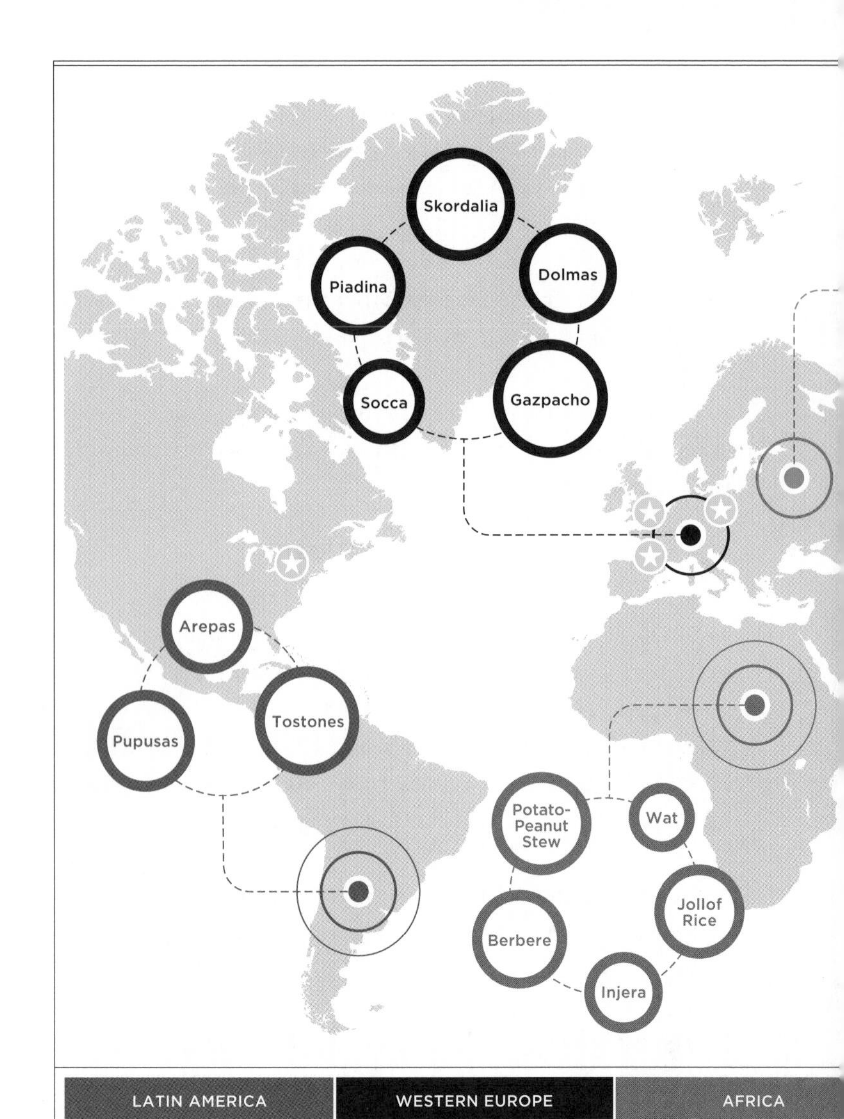

Skordalia
Piadina
Dolmas
Socca
Gazpacho
Arepas
Pupusas
Tostones
Potato-Peanut Stew
Wat
Jollof Rice
Berbere
Injera
LATIN AMERICA
WESTERN EUROPE
AFRICA

VEG-FRIENDLY FOOD AROUND THE WORLD

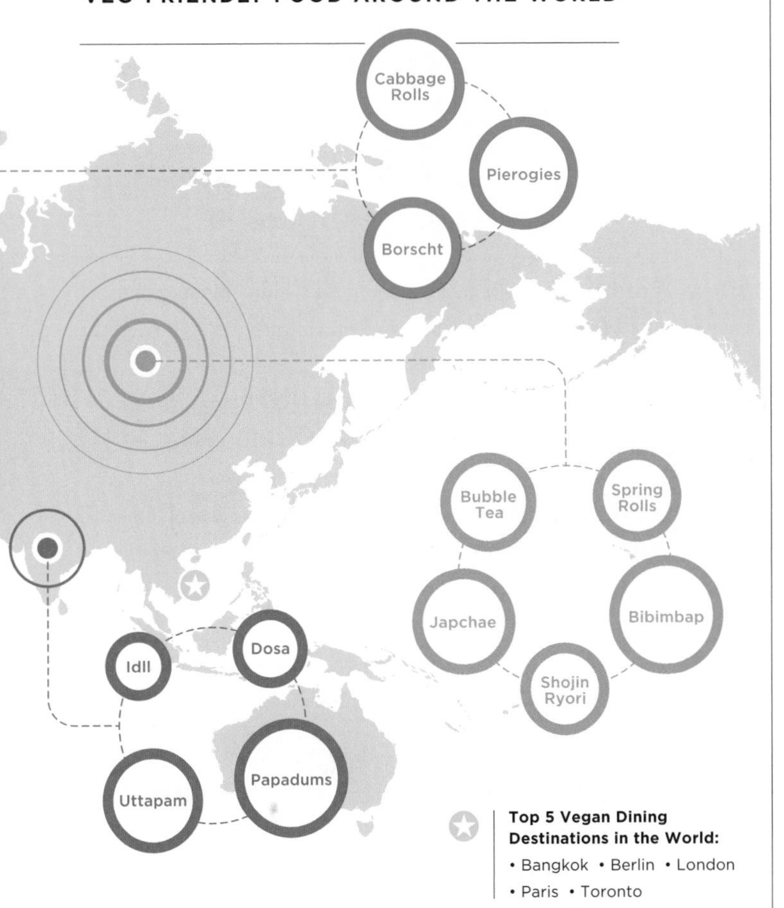

INDIA | EASTERN EUROPE | ASIA

WESTERN EUROPE

A good number of traditional dishes in Europe consist of freshly picked vegetables and grains doused in garlic and olive oil, which basically makes Europe a vegan buffet.

PIADINA: This toasty flatbread is a perfect street food from Italy. Grab one with fresh vegetables and pesto and you're all set.

SOCCA: Whether you get it in France or Italy, this chickpea-flour-based polenta is the perfect pick-me-up after a long day of sightseeing.

DOLMAS: No trip to Greece would be complete without a truckload of fresh, perfectly tart dolmas (grape leaves stuffed with rice).

SKORDALIA: Dip into this sumptuous spread with a freshly baked pita. Skordalia can be made from many things—the only real constants are garlic and olive oil—so look for potato-based versions.

GAZPACHO: Try this chilled tomato soup at tapas places in Spain. Cucumbers, red peppers, and tomatoes combine beautifully with olive oil and bread for a light, refreshing meal.

Pro Tip

Before you head out the door, check the website of the International Vegetarian Union (see Resources). This organization has members around the world and recommendations that can easily direct you to the best in-country finds.

INDIA

An incredible variety of vegetables simmered in the most exquisite blends of spices makes India a smorgasbord for vegans. Some dishes do contain ghee, or clarified butter, so ask about that.

DOSA: This crispy lentil-based pancake stuffed with aromatic potatoes and slathered in coconut chutney is almost as fun to eat as it is delicious.

PAPADUMS: These super-thin crackers infused with spices and dipped into chutneys provides a savory start to dinner.

UTTAPAM: A thicker pancake than the dosa, uttapam is savory with vegetables mixed in and comes with a selection of chutneys on the side.

IDLI: These round white cakes are usually served as part of breakfast, which is a pretty fantastic way to start the day. They don't have a ton of flavor on their own, but they pair perfectly with a spicy sambal.

Do	*Try fun new regional dishes!*
Don't	*Freak out if it turns out you've inadvertently consumed a tiny bit of something nonvegan. If you're doing your best, a little mishap doesn't erase all the delightful plant-based meals you regularly enjoy. This is actually just as true at home as it is on the road.*

TALK THE TALK

It's important to learn a few basic phrases in the language of the country you're visiting. In addition to "hello" and "thank you," figuring out how to say "I don't eat meat" or "I'm vegan" can be really helpful. One of the handiest ways to figure out how to say key phrases like this is the Google Translate app, which offers just about every language you could hope to need, as well as a vocal pronunciation for many of them. If you prefer a printed page to carry with you, visit MaxLearning.net and click on the Health tab. There you'll find V-Cards, which have key phrases such as "I'm vegan" and "No meat, please" in sixty-eight languages (the translations are sourced mostly from Google, but many are also edited by native speakers). Here's what "I'm vegan" looks like in a few of the most commonly traveled regions.

- Spanish: Soy vegano/a
- French: Je suis végétalien/végétalienne
- Italian: Sono vegano/a
- Japanese: 私はビーガンだ (Watashi wa bīganda)
- Chinese: 我是素食主义者 (Wǒ shì sùshí zhǔyì zhě)
- Arabic: أنا نبأنا نباتي (Ana nabati)
- Thai: ฉันมังสวิรัติ (Chạn mạngs̄wirạti)

LATIN AMERICA

Can you totally live happily on rice, beans, and fresh fruits and vegetables? Indeed you can, but there's much more to Latin cuisine than just the basic staples.

AREPAS: These corn cakes are popular in Latin America and can be filled with beans, vegetables, and slices of avocado for a satisfying sandwich.

TOSTONES: Is there anything better than plantains mashed, then fried, and served with either guacamole or chimichurri sauce? No, there isn't, and all of Latin America knows it.

PUPUSAS: These thick tortillas from El Salvador are typically stuffed with pork and cheese, but vegan versions filled with beans are also available.

TOP FIVE INTERNATIONAL DINING DESTINATIONS FOR VEGANS

Some cities really take it up a notch in terms of delicious vegan dining. The following five cities are more like never-ending buffets with some culture and sightseeing thrown in between eats.

- Bangkok
- Berlin
- London
- Paris
- Toronto

USA! USA! Dining Stateside

There's nary a corner of the United States that doesn't offer some insanely delicious foods, but there are also some real standout spots. Here are a few favorite vegan eating destinations. See Resources for more info.

LAS VEGAS

Surprise! Though the typical trip to Sin City might not be food focused, some absolutely world-class vegan cuisine is served there. Hotelier Steve Wynn tasked renowned vegan chef Tal Ronnen with creating showstopping menus for all of his properties' restaurants, including the room-service menus. From high-end Italian dining to inventive Asian cuisine, the variety and quality of dishes served makes Las Vegas a true desert oasis. And if you happen to venture off the Wynn grounds, there's Ronald's Donuts, an unassuming strip-mall doughnut shop where they serve some of the most phenomenally wonderful raised doughnuts of all time.

LOS ANGELES

As a native Northern Californian, it almost breaks my heart to say this, but Los Angeles has some fan-flipping-tastic vegan food. So many nonvegan places there have vegan offerings that you almost forget to look for exclusively vegan joints. You must, upon arriving at the airport, drive straight to M Café and get the M Chopped Salad and a bounty of pastries, then head to Shojin for dinner for the most mind-blowing sushi of all time. (Sushi isn't just limited to fish after all.

MUST-EATS IN AMERICA'S MOST VEGAN-FRIENDLY CITIES

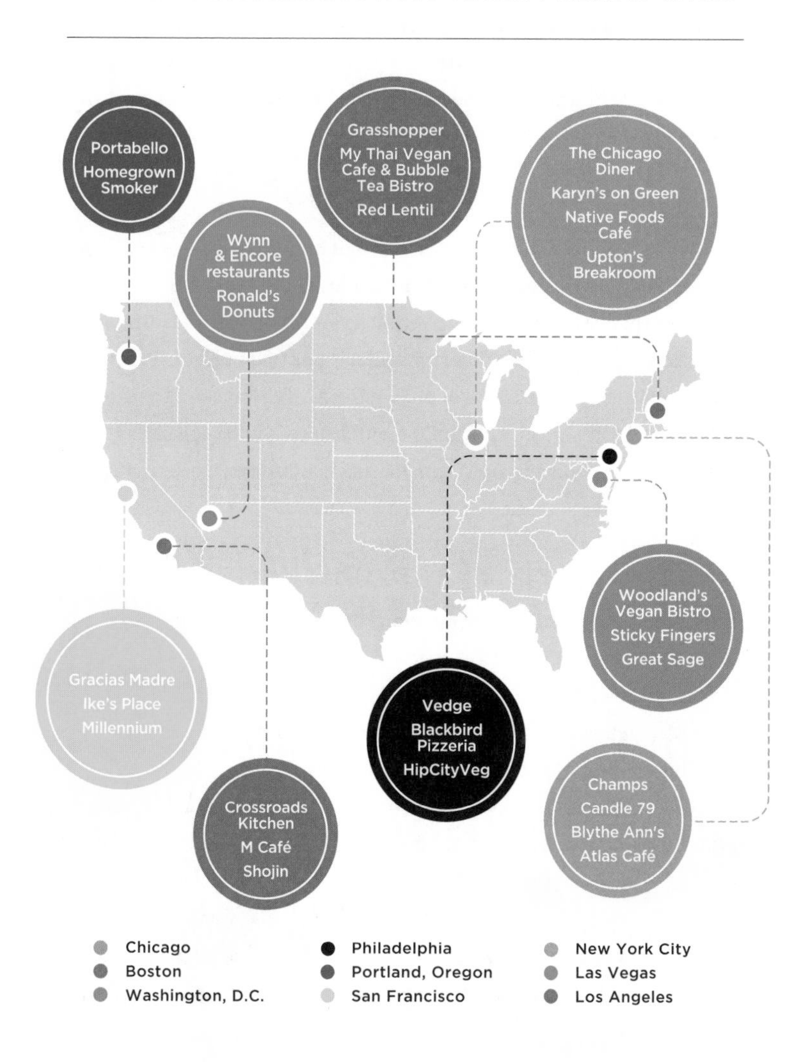

Shojin makes an incredible array of top-notch rolls filled with things like tempura pumpkin and spicy tempeh. Plus, the ramen is delicious.) The next day, make a reservation at Crossroads Kitchen, Tal Ronnen's incredible restaurant. Do not eat before you go. Order everything, especially the scaloppini. Be happy.

NEW YORK CITY

I know, I know. New York gets all the acclaim for basically everything, but seriously, it's a wonderland for vegans. There are more vegan restaurants than you could hope to visit even if you were visiting for a month. It also boasts my favorite vegan diner (Champs, in Brooklyn) and the best vegan ice cream shop (Blythe Ann's). Traveling as a vegan in New York City is a piece of cake—which you should get at Atlas Cafe, where you can find Vegan Treats cakes, aka the most amazing vegan cakes of all time.

PORTLAND, OREGON

For your unabashed inner glutton, Portland is where to take your loose-fitting pants. Vegan mac and cheese *inside* a burrito? Done. Plus, on the southeast side of town there's a vegan mini-mall, including a bakery, an adorable lifestyle shop, a grocery store, and a tattoo parlor. For fine dining, don't miss the phenomenal vegan Italian food at Portobello. The gnocchi is worth committing a felony for, in case you find yourself faced with that choice.

SAN FRANCISCO

Though it doesn't have the density of New York City or the sprawl of Los Angeles, San Francisco is a mighty fine place for yummy vegan food. Millennium is one of the best restaurants in the country, vegan or otherwise. It is high-end dining at its best, with a very involved menu, stunningly good cocktails, and a warm, inviting interior. In a city known for its Mexican food, Gracias Madre is a standout, and not only because it's vegan and organic. The plantain tacos are heavenly. Ike's Place is a mini-chain that isn't totally vegan but offers the most decadent sandwiches of all time (the Vegan Pilgrim has Tofurky, cranberry sauce, vegan cheese, and hot sauce), all served on rolls with Ike's signature Dirty Sauce, which sounds gross but tastes like garlicky perfection.

COMPLETELY VEGAN GETAWAYS

Where to go if you're in the States and don't want to have to bother asking whether there will be almond milk for your morning coffee? Check out one of these totally vegan and very wonderful places to stay.

DEER RUN BED & BREAKFAST, BIG PINE KEY, FLORIDA

Hoping for the tropics but not keen on leaving the country? Good news—we have Florida. The sandy beaches right out the front door of Deer Run will cure what ails you. (And yes, deer have been seen on the property—the owners even put up a deer cam for fans of fawns!)

THE GINGER CAT BED & BREAKFAST, ROCK STREAM, NEW YORK

If you can't resist the call of fall foliage, this is the place for you. The Ginger Cat is in the rolling hills of upstate New York and offers homey, casual rooms.

THE STANFORD INN, MENDOCINO, CALIFORNIA

Do in-room fireplaces, acres of gardens, and an amazing restaurant sound good to you? (If not, definitely do not book a stay here.) The Stanford Inn is one of the country's most renowned inns, and its restaurant, The Ravens, is equally impressive. The brunch menu is the stuff of legends, and the views (the inn sits snugly on a coastal hill in Northern California) are spectacular.

Where To?

Aside from just scouting out the best restaurants around the globe and basing your vacations on where you'd most like to eat (not that there's anything wrong with this approach, mind you!), deciding on the kind of trip you'd like to take will make planning easier. Want to spend your summer biking through Europe? Surfing a tropical shore? Caravanning through India? Here are a few suggestions for ways to spend your precious vacation time. See Resources for more info.

ANIMAL SANCTUARIES, AKA THE BEST PLACES ON EARTH

There is absolutely nothing like getting up close to a farm animal. They're so sweet and strange; so visually familiar but physically completely unknown. The first time I visited a sanctuary it was for a fund-raising gala, and we enjoyed a lovely dinner all dressed up, walking in heels through the barns. There was an enormous Brahman bull that was all business in an open arena, and in a cozy little barn there were the springiest baby goats. Just like you'd see with dogs or cats, within moments of being around these truly odd-looking animals (they just look completely different when they're inches from your face instead of in photographs—or, grossly, disassembled and wrapped in butcher paper), it became obvious that each one was an individual and that each had a distinct personality. As with most experiences in life, you can't know how insanely sweet and soft a huge cow is until you've gone up and rubbed her face and silky shoulders. That's where farm animal sanctuaries come in. If you haven't been, go. Farm Sanctuary, Woodstock Farm Animal Sanctuary, and The Gentle Barn are three of the best known in the country, but there are many smaller ones dotted across the States. Many have B and Bs attached or nearby, and because they need room for the animals to roam, the majority are located in the country, which makes for a perfect excuse to get some fresh air.

WHY ANIMAL SANCTUARIES ARE THE BEST

Getting up close and personal with sweet animals
+
Enjoying sunshine and fresh air
+
Meeting the dedicated, hardworking staff
=
A truly memorable vacation experience

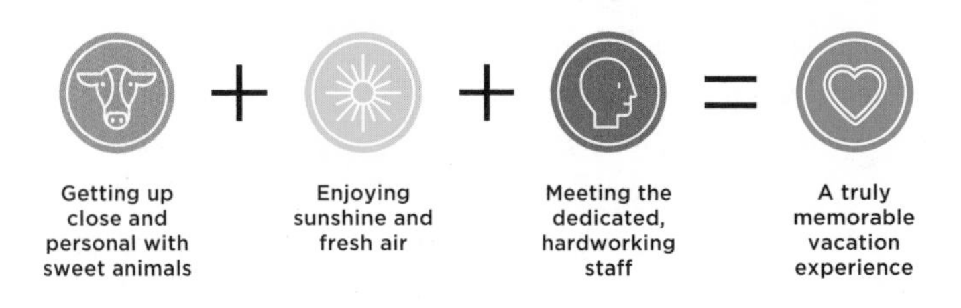

CRUISIN'

Each year the Holistic Holiday at Sea takes off on a Caribbean tour from Florida and makes stops in ports usually including Puerto Rico, the Bahamas, and St. Maarten. As the name implies, the cruise has a health focus and serves as a conference-at-sea with presentations from leading nutrition experts, yoga classes, and healthy fare. If you're looking to boast about being "on a boat" to friends, this might be the perfect way to do it.

GUIDED GROUPS

Sometimes you just want someone else to do the planning so you can kick back and not make decisions while on vacation. A number of organizations offer vegan-specific tour packages. VegVoyages is the best known and takes tourists through India, Indonesia, Laos, Thailand, and Malaysia. VegVoyages arranges itineraries (sights to see, where to eat and stay, and transportation) for each destination and leads groups of travelers through the country. Tierno Tours offers a similar experience in Italy.

AHHH, SPAS

Do we need to talk about why spas are great? Because they're really, really great, especially if you're into things like a beautiful, peaceful location where people are super nice to you and do wonderful, scrubby things to your tired body. Going for a spa vacation is never a bad idea, and many of them cater to vegans, so you can unwind without worrying that your salt scrub has sneaky animal ingredients. The best resource for finding the perfect vegan-friendly spa is Google, since there are a ton throughout the States and around the globe, including Ten Thousand Waves in Santa Fe, New Mexico, and Haramara Retreat in Sayulita, Mexico.

THREE INCREDIBLE INTERNATIONAL SPAS

If you're going all in for rest, relaxation, and travel, these three places in stunning locations take relaxation to an entirely new level (see Resources).

- El Remanso Lodge, Puerto Jimenez, Costa Rica
- The Farm, Lipa City, Philippines
- Five Elements, Mambal, Bali, Indonesia

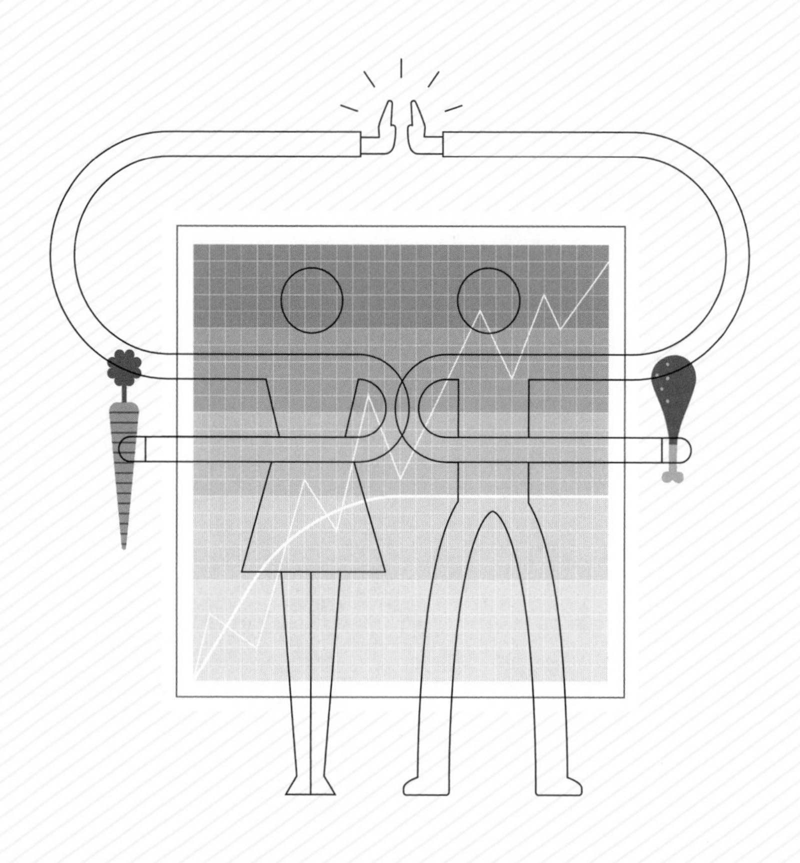

5

MANNERS

DON'T BE A JERK

"Whatever you are, be a good one."

—ABRAHAM LINCOLN

What's the first thing that comes to mind when you hear the word *vegan*? Go ahead, be honest. Is it the ever-delightful Ellen DeGeneres? Or is the image more of that guy at the party who berates you for serving crackers that aren't 100 percent organic, GMO free, soy free, gluten free, palm oil free, and lichen free? If a persnickety pesterer or a meddlesome misanthrope is what you equate the word *vegan* with, I have great news. You totally get to change the way people think about vegans. See, when we're mean jerks about enjoying our plant-based lifestyle, people think vegans are mean jerks. When we are nice, decent humans who happen to forgo animal products, people think vegans are nice, decent humans. It's nutty how that works, right? In this chapter, we'll look at some of the situations in which our niceness and decency can be put to the test and how it's totally possible to maintain your sanity while fielding all sorts of questions, jokes, and (on occasion) downright insults.

Manners, Mildly

There are many reasons the Superman story is fantastic, although etiquette isn't usually the first thing that comes to mind when people talk about the Man of Steel. But the thing is, Clark Kent's dorky, mild-mannered, genuinely nice persona is one of the things that allows us native Earth residents to relate to him so easily: you get to cheer for the underdog (especially while he's pining for Lois Lane) while simultaneously celebrating the successes of the überhero. The most effective advocates for any group, lifestyle, or cause are people like this: they're genuine and kind, and their integrity is something that others want to emulate. Where's all this going? It's very common for people to be curious about your veganism (aka, asking roughly 8.7 zillion questions), and it's also common for people to say thoughtlessly insensitive things. Figuring out how to navigate social situations as Mr. Kent would (that is, nicely) is a lifelong project.

SPONTANEOUS COMBUSTION:

THE HIDDEN DANGER OF VEGANISM

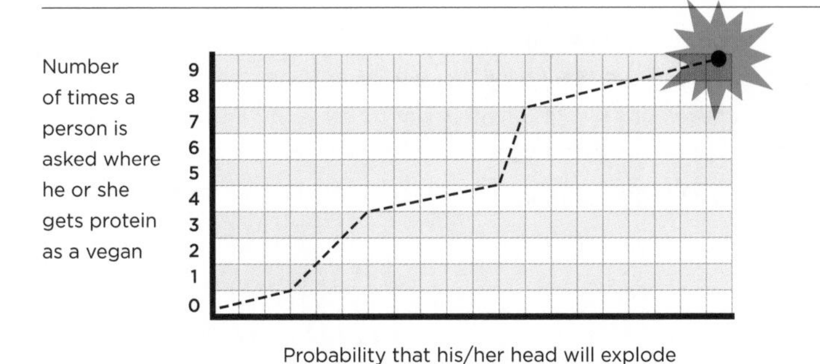

DEALING WITH THE DIFFICULT

Here are a few of the types of people you are likely to encounter. (Of course, none of my friends or family members has ever done anything like this, because they are all perfect. Obviously.) For each example, pick the option for dealing with this person that reflects the best manners.

1. The Well-Meaning but Uninformed Parents Who Think You're About to Drop Dead from Malnutrition

OPTION 1: Every time your dad mentions that you're not getting enough iron, rip open your shirt, stomp through the house, and scream, "HULK SMASH! HULK SMASH!" This will prove your brawn and allay his fears.

OPTION 2: Do your research! Get your blood tested to see where your nutrient levels are, and if there are any that need bolstering, consult your doctor about how to do so without eating pork rinds.

They hound you because they care, right? Even so, hearing that you're constantly on the verge of wasting away to nothing and dropping dead from lack of sausage likely isn't good for a healthy parent-child relationship, no matter the ages of the parents or children. Prove your knowledge and responsibility, not your Bruce Banner–like freak-out ability.

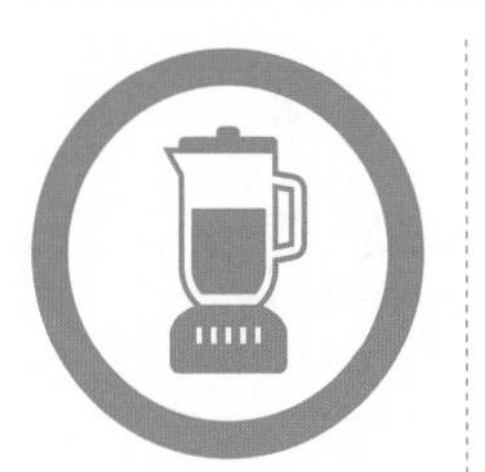

2. The Jokey Uncle Who Asks at Every Single Meal If You Want Some Butter on Your Bread/Some Cheese on Your Pasta/Some Meaty Gravy on Your Mashed Potatoes

OPTION 1: Tell him you'd like all of those things. Put them in a blender together, then drink them through a straw, just to gross him out.

OPTION 2: Say, "No, thanks."

"No, thanks" is one of two key phrases for life (the other, for the record, is "Yes, thanks").

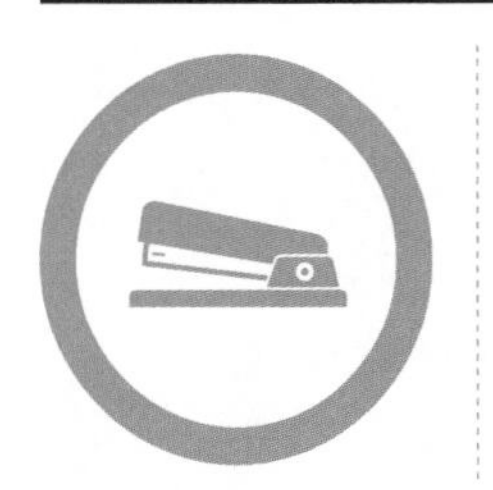

3. The Flat-Out Rude Co-Worker Who Stops by Your Desk Every Day at Lunch to Eat His Turkey Sandwich and Berate You, Saying That Vegans Are a Lowlier Subset of Humans

OPTION 1: Go to work on a Saturday and bring as much plastic wrap as you can carry. Wrap every single thing on his desk, including the stapler, keyboard, mouse, binder clips, and his coffee mug, then, for the grand finale, wrap his chair to his desk. While you're wrapping, toss a few slices of Tofurky into the layers so that come Monday, he arrives to a cold-cut-covered mess. Make especially sure to wrap the scissors in a few extra layers so they are completely unreachable.

OPTION 2: Ask him politely to stop. If it keeps up, report him to HR. That's why the department exists.

You'll quickly develop a sort of sixth sense for when someone legitimately has an interest in your diet and might want to adjust his own eating habits, and when he is being a straight-up jerk.

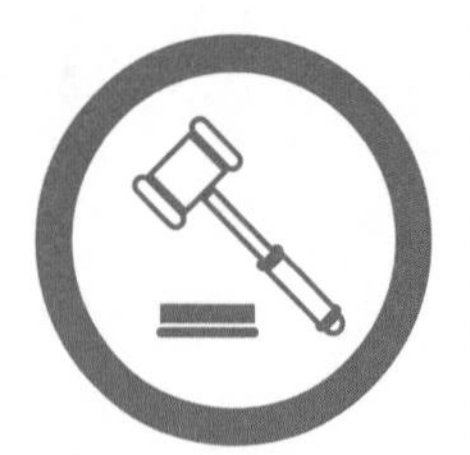

4. The Overzealous Vegan Who Judges You for Not Being Vegan Enough

OPTION 1: Actually, there's only one option here. Ignore people like this. How you live is, frankly, not their business, and it makes way more sense to encourage people in what they are doing to make the world better than to hound them for what they are not doing. The fact that we can't do everything doesn't mean we should do nothing. (Oh, you're not also saving babies in Africa and volunteering at the local animal shelter and reading to the elderly and building latrines in Cambodia and staffing a soup kitchen all while working full-time and caring for your family? Sheesh, you lazy punk, what *do* you do with your time?)

Do	*Have a two-sentence summary of why you're giving plant-based eating a try at the ready. This will save tons of time.*
Don't	*Try to transmit to someone every bit of information you have about veganism and the multitudinous reasons it's amazing all at once. Yes, there really are many, many great reasons to eat plants, but spewing them all in a big info dump doesn't make for an amazing conversation.*

5. The 500th Person Who Asks "Where Do You Get Your Protein?" Plus All the People Who Ask the Very Same Question Thereafter

OPTION 1: Smile kindly and reply, "Plants."

OPTION 2: Don't smile. Gruffly growl out, "Plants, dum-dum."

See what I did there? The right answer was Option 2 for all of the other examples, but then, blammo, out of nowhere, for number five it switched. Tricky, I know. Basically, the thing you want to do anytime your choices are challenged is the same: respond with understanding and kindness. It's very likely that if you're reading this book you haven't been vegan your entire life, so helping people understand why you've made this choice (even if you make it every third meal) is a great opportunity to share your experience. Plus, really, no one likes a Rude Gus in any situation, so don't be that guy!

Meet This Vegan: DENNIS KUCINICH

Remember that time when a vegan almost became president of the United States? Well, maybe that's slightly overstating it, but Dennis Kucinich did run for the highest office in the land twice, not to mention serving an impressive sixteen years as a congressman representing his home state of Ohio. Dennis and his wife, Elizabeth, are indefatigable campaigners for animals, using their position in the media to garner attention for the environmental benefits of living a vegan lifestyle, among other important causes.

WHEN SOMEONE IS SUPER RUDE ABOUT YOUR DIET

Yup, this is going to happen. No matter how kind, compassionate, and reasonable you are, there's something about saying you're vegan that brings out a strange side in others. Some people will be awed and interested, others completely indifferent, and still others will immediately go into the many reasons they could never be vegan. Note that you didn't ask them whether *they* could but simply stated that *you* are. When someone is rude, shake it off. It does the animals, the planet, and your health less good to have someone think that all vegans are angst-ridden, argumentative misanthropes than to calmly respond, "Ah, well, it's been working nicely for me," and leave it at that.

WHEN YOU'VE BEEN RUDE

Apologize. It doesn't matter whether or not your veganism was part of the offense. If you've been rude, it's probably best to own up to it and try to set things right than to be remembered as a jerk, right?

Entertaining . . . and Being Entertained

You know, Emily Post had the right idea. Maybe we don't all need to use spoons in ascending size order, but a good portion of society could use a primer on being polite. If you are very lucky, people will invite you to their homes for dinner, they will want to celebrate holidays with you, and they'll call you up for cocktail parties. The biggest worry about going to or hosting social functions as a vegan should be the same thing it is for every single other person on the planet: trying to chat someone up while having something huge and gross stuck in your teeth—not the convenience factor of your dietary choices.

EASY VEGAN DINNER PARTY MENU

Totally unsure of where to start when planning a plant-based feast? If you're having between four and ten people over, these kinds of dishes scale up and down easily and go well together. Look online for recipes, using these suggestions as starting points.

- **Starters:** Crackers, white bean dip with rosemary, olives
- **Salad:** Fennel, arugula, avocado, and toasted pine nuts with olive oil, cracked pepper, and sea salt
- **Soup:** Tomato and rice
- **Main:** Pizza with caramelized onions, fennel, and capers
- **Side:** Roasted broccoli with garlic and red pepper flakes
- **Dessert:** Creamy Chocolate Pie (page 202)

Do	*Let the host know that although you're sure his recipe for beef tartare is fantastic, you're really looking forward to his spring rolls.*
Don't	*Go to a party starving when you're not sure what will be served. Chances are you're there to enjoy the company of the other guests, and it's a bonus if the food ends up being great. If you go without anything in your stomach, you'll just end up getting drunk and saying something embarrassing before you've even had a chance to see if there's anyone there you might like to get to know.*

HOW TO BEHAVE WHEN YOU ARE A GUEST

Step one here is the same as anywhere else: be nice! Call your host ahead of time and offer to bring a dish. A good friend will likely already know what you do and don't eat. For new friends, let them know that you're super happy to contribute something to the meal, and if vegan cooking is completely new to your host and he or she wants to make something just for you, offer resources for recipes. No matter what the host says, show up with a bottle of wine or bubbly. If you're served a bowl of oatmeal with soy sauce while everyone else enjoys filet mignon, genuinely thank the host for making you something special. While people are milling around after dinner enjoying coffee and conversation, sneak into the kitchen and do the dishes.

HOW TO BE A GOOD VEGAN HOST

That whole "do unto others" thing definitely applies here. Make sure you know about any allergies or restrictions your guests have and then serve something really deeply, insanely yummy. For groups of mixed preferences, it's best to stick to dishes that are naturally vegan (or nearly so) instead of attempting to re-create everyone's favorite meat-based dishes with stand-in products. Is a Tofurky sandwich with avocado, lettuce, and a perfectly spicy mustard a delicious lunch option? Yes. Is it going to wow guests and entice them to return to your gatherings? Probably not. Try something simple and flavorful, such as a platter of pesto pasta with a vibrant salad or a big pot of spicy red curry with tofu and vegetables. Sushi-making is a great party option because guests can personalize rolls to their tastes and everyone has fun in the process.

PARTY TIME

A flowchart for successful party planning.

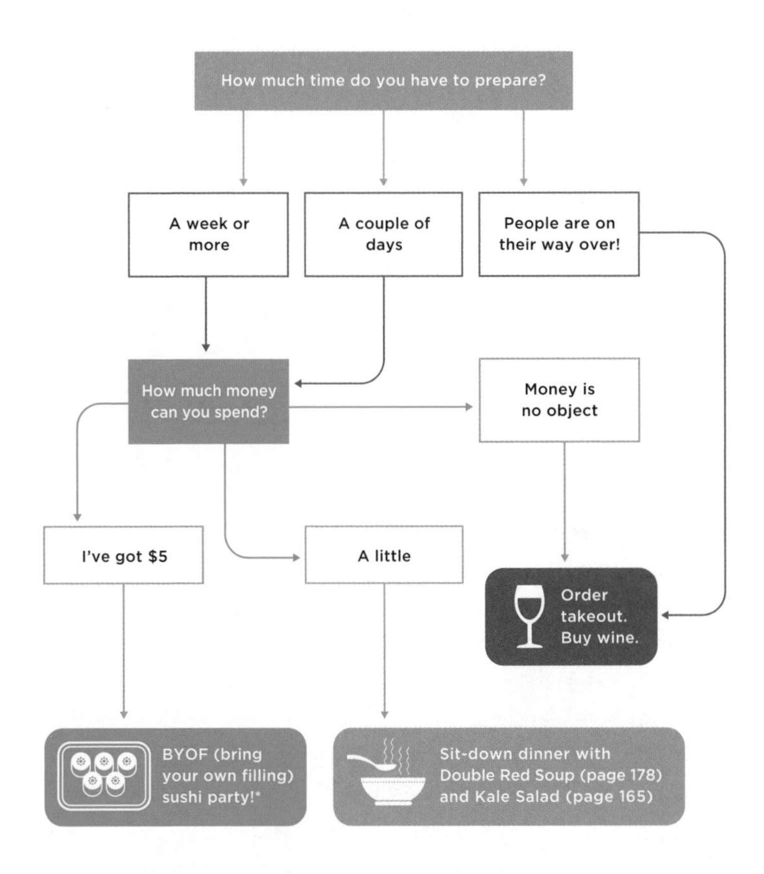

*Psst! These fillings are always good: roasted peanuts, avocado, fishless tuna with hearts of palm, roasted yams, Rice Krispies, cucumbers, carrots

HOW TO BE A GOOD HOST TO VEGANS

If you are not vegan (and if you're reading this book, you may be considering it but not yet committed to the idea) and you're having a couple of plant eaters over for dinner, thank you! That's awfully nice. As with most dinner parties (or cocktail parties, or birthday parties, or any other excuse to get together and have fun), if these people are good friends of yours, you'll likely already know what kinds of foods they enjoy most. If you don't know your guests terribly well, plan a menu with at least one option that works for everyone. If you're serving a roast beef main course, it would be considerate to make sure that there's a vegan grain dish or casserole for a side, so that the vegans will still be full (see page 140 re the dangers of serving alcohol to people with empty stomachs). Of course, if you're making the whole menu vegan in deference to your guests, (a) you should be inducted into the hosting hall of fame, and (b) as you would with any guests, don't make this dinner party the time to go way beyond your culinary comfort zone. Make something that you've made a million times and know will be tasty to everyone's palate. If it's a casual evening, fajitas are some of the easiest, most successful vegan mains on the planet. Warm tortillas, lightly sautéed bell peppers and onions, savory beans, rice, salsa, and avocado? Heaven.

Do	*Serve dishes that you enjoy eating—it's your party, after all.*
Don't	*Veer too deeply into unknown culinary territory. Perfect your dairy-free three-cheese lasagne before debuting it at a dinner party.*

Meet This Vegan: MAYIM BIALIK

It would be really easy to make a crack about Mayim Bialik blossoming into a vegan advocate, but it feels a bit cheap considering that the hilarious actress is also a neuroscientist and an author. Basically, she's the total package. Funny, smart, and classy, Bialik went vegan after reading Jonathan Safran Foer's *Eating Animals* in 2010 and has been a sprout stumper ever since. She starred in a retro-style campaign for PETA that encouraged fans to protect their families from food-borne illness by tossing out meat and penned a vegan family-themed cookbook to follow her first book, *Beyond the Sling*, about attachment parenting.

NOT EVERY ACTIVITY HAS TO INVOLVE FOOD

It can take a really long time to learn the following lesson, especially if you grew up in a family that enjoys eating and entertaining, but it is well worth the effort: not every meal has to be an event, and not every event has to be a meal. Sure, if you're eating anyway, sharing that time with a friend is often more satisfying than hunching over your laptop as an endless stream of online shows plays incessantly. But does that mean the only option for seeing the people in your life is to invite them for brunch, lunch, or dinner? Turns out it's not. Anything you might

Pro Tip

Serving pasta but want it to feel fancy and elegant? Switch out your regular shape for gnocchi—most store-bought brands are vegan—and top with a smooth sauce (chunky sauces such as puttanesca work better with ridged pasta so that the sauce can stick to the starch).

think to do that isn't centered on food is fair game for friend time. See a movie, take in a play, hike around your local wilderness area, go for a run or a bike ride, explore a museum, hit up your favorite bookstore, lounge in the sun, pet each and every last dog at the dog park—really, there are so many ways to see friends that don't involve the yes-we-can-go-to-your-favorite-steak-house-for-dinner-and-I'll-just-order-the-baked-potato-again conundrum.

It sometimes, though not always, happens that going vegan makes it uncomfortable to watch others eating meat. If this is true for you, suggest to your pals that you do something fun together, instead of eating something fun together. If you really need to sit down for a good chat—the kind usually conducted over a long dinner with drinks—meet up at a coffee house instead.

L'Amour

When a person decides to live by a set of principles, it can affect his or her dating life. In matters of the heart, following your heart matters. Whether you decide that you're going to wear only blue shirts from this day forward or you adjust your diet to better reflect your values, dating someone who is supportive of you and your passions is pretty imperative.

DATING DELIGHTFULLY

Once you swear off meat on your plate, do you need to limit your potential dating pool to only the herbivorous? Nah. Do you—just like every other single person on the planet—want to go out with people you like and who like you? If someone is a jerk about your veganism (say, every time you go out, she jokes about how you're eating rabbit food, makes

BOOS TO ZOOS

There are a few nonfood activities that you might want to reconsider: the ones at which animals are exploited for humans' entertainment. Zoos, circuses, and marine mammal parks are unfortunately rife with abuse. Though many people see these places as havens for animals that would otherwise be unable to cope in their natural habitats, this is not the case with animal parks. From cruel handlers beating elephants with bull hooks to force them into performing to dolphins being trapped in tiny tanks until they literally go insane from not being able to engage in their natural behaviors, the fates of animals used to entertain humans are grim at best. It's worth considering whether the tiger jumping through a flaming hoop would do so if not for an intense conditioning process. Some zoos have worked to bring species on the brink of extinction back to health, and some rescue animals from private collections or animal parks, but then there are also those that routinely sell their animals off for exotic meats—not exactly a conservation effort. As with anything, it's a good idea to do your research before supporting something (a zoo, a restaurant, an artist) with your money.

mean comments to your friends, or belittles this thing that you really, deeply care about), that's a pretty big red flag. Of course, it would be just as big a red flag if the person you were dating was a total jerk about your hair color or your height. Basically, if you're into actually liking the person you're dating, it's probably best not to go out with a jerk. Having shared ethics when it comes to animals isn't a panacea for all relationship ills, but it does serve as a connection point.

SHOULD I DATE THIS PERSON?

When picking a partner, consider these categories. Being vegan isn't the only thing to look for in a partner.

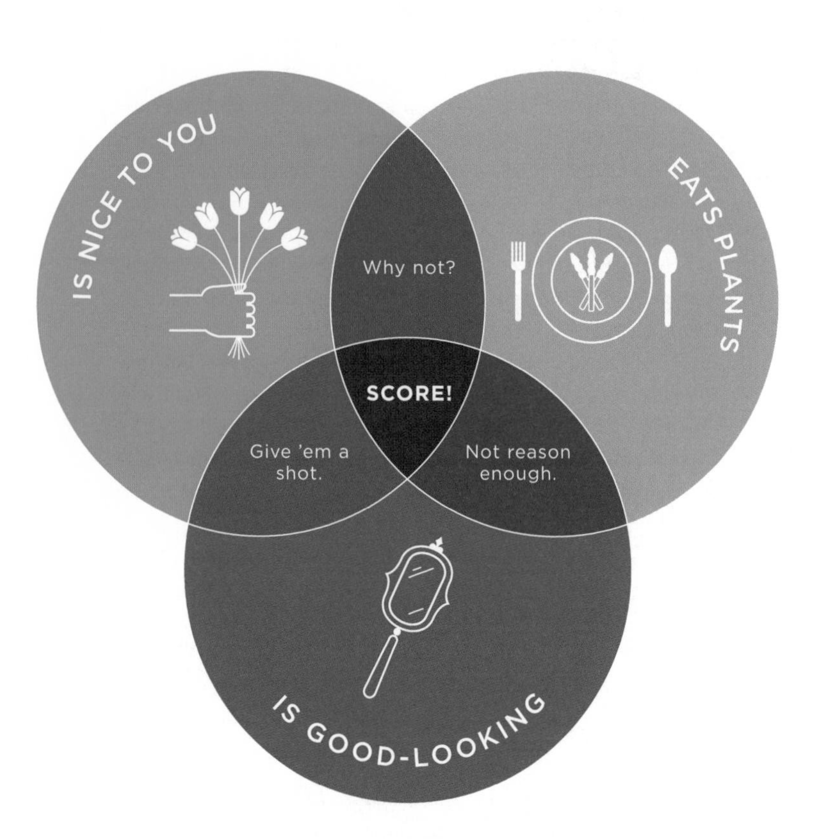

Here's a handy quiz to decide whether someone is worth dating. Choose the option(s) that must be met:

Option 1: The person is genuinely nice to you, treats you well, and is fun to be around.

Option 2: The person eats plants.

Option 3: Both of the above.

If you picked either 1 or 3, bravo! Option 2 just isn't enough on its own. Plus, it's very likely that if you start dating someone who usually eats meat, and you're a decent enough partner to cook for her once in a while, then she'll be eating vegan more frequently than if you weren't dating. Win-win!

But if the idea of seeing meat eaten in front of you is off-putting, then you will likely want to stick to dating fellow veggie-eaters, since cringing every time you go out for dinner does not a happy relationship make. If you have become a sworn plant person but are open to the idea of dating outside that realm, just remember to make sure that both you and your partner are happy with the arrangement. Maybe you cook for each other once in a while, and she makes you your favorite vegan lasagne. Maybe you both cook for yourselves, but you sit down together to eat so that you can still share in mealtime bonding. Whatever arrangement you come to, when things get serious, it's important to communicate what you are and are not comfortable with so that there aren't surprises along the way or you feel like your values are compromised.

MARRIAGE MATERIAL

Getting hitched? Good for you! Assuming here that you've found someone who brings more joy than strife to your life, mazel tov. If you want to have a vegan wedding, check out Rose Pedals Vegan Weddings (see Resources), an online resource for vendors, stories of vegan wedding successes, and etiquette tips. But what to do if the nuptials are not yours? If you're a guest at a wedding, treat it the way you would any event that's beyond your control. If the couple offers a vegan meal option, that's awesome. If not, pack a couple extra Clif bars in your bag or pocket, and have fun.

Do	*Make sure to eat enough bread that you don't accidentally get super drunk and make a total moron out of yourself. Most rolls are vegan, so go to town.*
Don't	*Hound the couple incessantly before the wedding to ensure that they'll have food for you. The day is about them, not you, and frankly they probably have enough to deal with as the day approaches.*

OH, BABY!

As we all know, there's a pretty well established trajectory of love, marriage, and then a certain carriage. Is this what everyone wants? No. However, if you are of the procreation persuasion, is it possible as a vegan? Absolutely. Again, the plant-based diet is safe and healthy for people of all ages, including pregnant women, breast-feeding mothers, and infants. Many pregnant vegan women notice that, much like what happens when any woman begins to share the news of her baby, her friends and family suddenly become experts in prenatal care. The best

IF YOU REALLY LOVED ME . . .

Is there ever an end to this phrase that doesn't screw things up? You know whether or not the person you're with really loves you—just don't kid yourself. Joining you in veganism isn't a measure of anyone's feelings for you, but it can be something that you introduce the person to and that he or she then decides to try out. Trying to get someone to go vegan "for you" is flat-out dumb. Imagine any time someone has tried to tell you to do something you weren't keen on doing. Inside us all lives a permanent four-year-old who just wants to scream, "You can't make me!" and run away. And even if your guy or gal is superhumanly docile and accepting of authority, veganism is a choice that should be made for oneself. Otherwise, that person's commitment to plant-eating is doomed as soon as the relationship dies (and let's be honest, out of all the people you've dated, how many of them have become your one and only for life?).

defense against the sometimes-inquisitive, sometimes-downright-pushy interrogations of loved ones is to read up on exactly the kinds of nutrients that pregnancy requires. Like all pregnant women, vegan moms-to-be do need to pay specific attention to their diets to make sure that the baby grows up healthy, but it is absolutely doable. Here are three books you'll want to read the moment the pregnancy test turns blue.

- *The Everything Vegan Pregnancy Book*, by Reed Mangels
- *Vegan for Life*, by Jack Norris and Virginia Messina
- *Vegan Pregnancy Survival Guide*, by Sayward Rebhal

Hello, Holidays

No matter what your eating preferences are, the holidays can be a mixed bag of excitement, stress, cocktails, cinnamon rolls, and wrapping paper. Keeping yourself sane when family descends from out of town, every night is packed with cookie baking and present wrapping, and there is more celebrating to be done than any human is actually capable of can be a bit taxing. Plus, many traditional holiday foods aren't naturally vegan, so it can take a little creativity to enjoy the same foods you grew up making for special occasions.

KEEP THE PEACE

When family that doesn't spend a ton of time together is suddenly thrown into the same house for somewhat extended periods of time, tempers can run high, emotions can come up, and drinkers can get drunk. Instead of reverting to a petulant teenager's mentality when faced with the holidays—and an extra level of dietary scrutiny—adopt an attitude of gratitude. Sure, it sounds a little cheesy. But it also is incredibly helpful. Be thankful for the opportunity to see your family, and thankful for the chance to share delicious plant-based options with everyone at the table; it's a great way to get through the yearly inquisition from Nana about why you don't eat brisket anymore. Remember, everyone is probably also asking your sister why she hasn't gotten married yet or asking your mother why she decided to serve buffet instead of family-style this year. Basically, everyone has something that is worthy of familial scrutiny. So grin and bear it.

HOLIDAY SURVIVAL GUIDE

The key elements to making the holidays work!

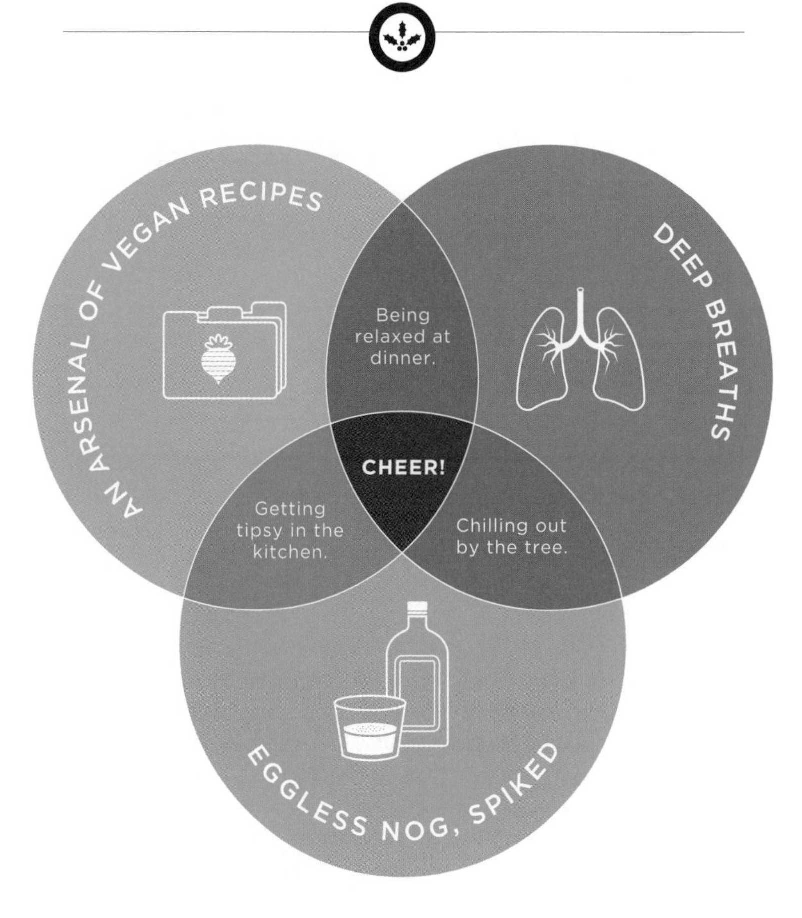

MAKING THE FOODS

Half the fun of the holidays is turning the kitchen into a sweets factory. For many recipes, substituting vegan butter is all you need to do for perfect pies and cookies, but what about more complicated dishes? Not sure where to turn for reliable, just-like-Grandma-made-but-veganized recipes for the holidays? Look no further. These cookbooks cover all the major holidays, as well as a slew of lesser-known ones, and are sure to keep your family and guests fed and festive.

- *Celebrate Vegan,* by Dynise Balcavage
- *Gluten-Free and Vegan Holidays,* by Jennifer Katzinger
- *Vegan Holiday Kitchen,* by Nava Atlas

Meet This Vegan: CASEY AFFLECK

Soft-spoken actor Casey Affleck has enjoyed the vegan lifestyle for more than a decade. In a video interview with PETA, Affleck says that when he first went vegan he found it difficult to go out to restaurants and find cruelty-free clothing and accessories like belts, but the longer he's lived this way, the easier it's become, in large part thanks to the availability of anything you could want on the Internet. Veganism is part of Affleck's family too: he's married to lifelong vegan Summer Phoenix, Joaquin's sister. Affleck has worked with PETA on campaigns condemning the dehorning of cows, the abuses animals suffer on factory farms, and leghold traps (used in hunting).

GRIEF-FREE GIFTS

If someone wants to give you a present, that's fantastic. It does sometimes happen that you'll get something for the holidays that doesn't mesh with your ethics, which can present a bit of an etiquette dilemma. When Aunt Alexandra gives you a lovely cashmere sweater (yep, that's made from goats!), you basically have three options:

RETURN IT: Step one: say thank you. That's the first thing to do with any gift. If there's a gift receipt included, it's implied that the giver is leaving the fate of the sweater up to you. If there's no gift receipt but you are very close to Auntie A, ask her how she'd like you to handle it. Explain, "I'm so touched that you got this for me, and I don't want that thoughtfulness to go to waste. Since I don't wear wool, would you like to return it, or should I pass it along to someone at work who'll love it?" This suggestion leads us to your next option.

REGIFT IT: Step one is still saying thank you, in case that wasn't clear. If you don't see this particular aunt very often, and it will likely cause her stress to learn that her gift doesn't work with your ethics, you might consider just regifting it (yes, the "person" you give it to could be your local homeless shelter or Goodwill).

WEAR IT: Nearly every vegan on the planet has some nonvegan items in his closet, whether they're from prevegan days or secondhand shops or gifts. What you do with nonvegan items is a choice, just like all the other small choices we make throughout the day. A situation like this is an opportunity to have a conversation with your aunt about why you don't buy this kind of thing for yourself, as she might not be aware of the process that animals go through when they're used for clothing. Just be sure your actions align with your actual ethics—for instance, if you wouldn't buy a leather bag, does it make sense to wear a cashmere sweater?

THE PERFECT GIFT

There are so many incredible vegan products on the market these days; finding something to give that is free of animal products is easier than ever. Here are a few ideas for the vegans on your gift list.

ADOPT AN ANIMAL: Most animal sanctuaries offer gift adoptions, which isn't the commitment it sounds like. You don't come home with a baby turkey, but your donation goes to supporting a specific animal at the sanctuary. Check out Woodstock Farm Animal Sanctuary, Farm Sanctuary, or the Gentle Barn (see Resources).

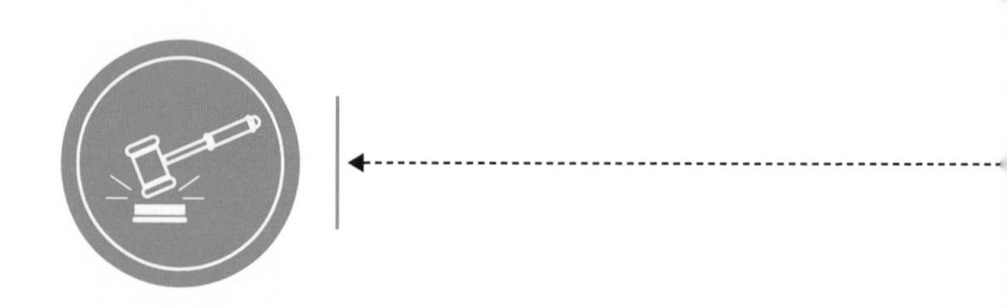

DONATE SOME DOLLARS: If there's an organization that your favorite vegan loves, give it some money! Groups such as Compassion over Killing, Mercy for Animals, and the Humane Society of the United States (see Resources) do amazing work for animals and depend on donations.

MAKE IT MICRO: There are so many great micro-loan and crowd-funding sites these days, which means that there's a ton of opportunity to give some money to people who are doing creative, interesting projects to help animals. Whether it's a baker who's looking to buy more equipment on Kickstarter or a loan to a fledgling animal sanctuary on Kiva, giving a gift in honor of someone is a solid option. Plus, does anyone actually need another tchotchke?

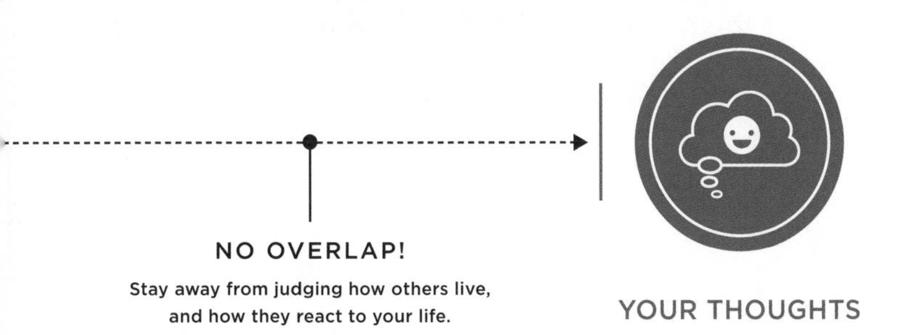

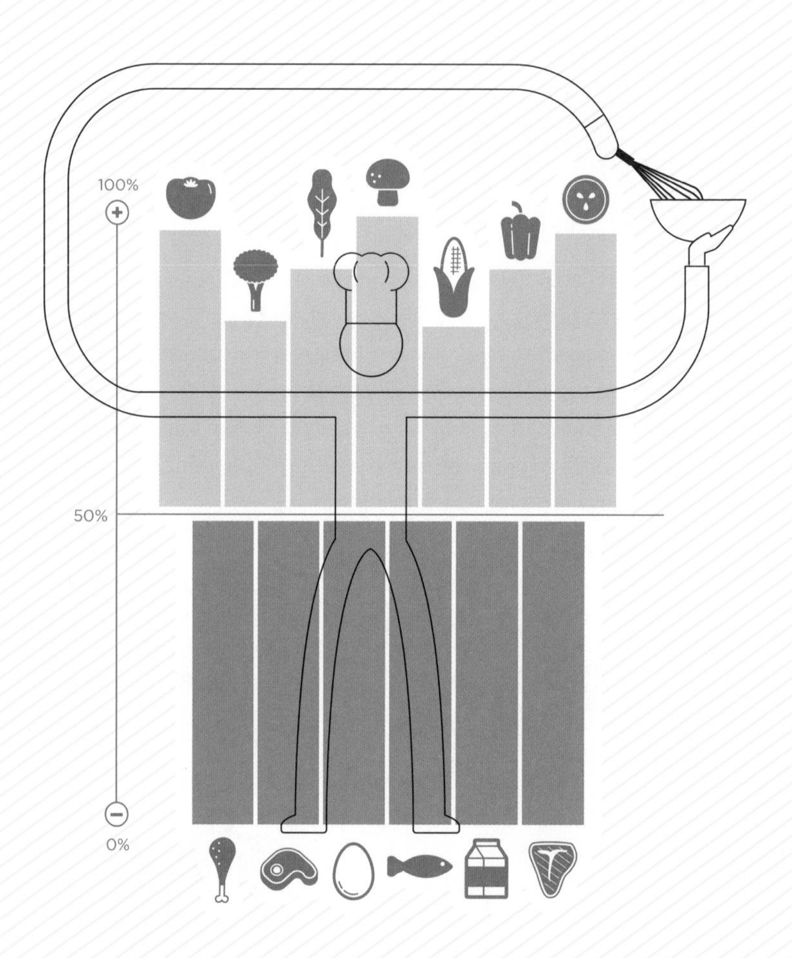
100%
50%
0%

6

THE RECIPES

GET INTO THE KITCHEN

"Humor keeps us alive. Humor and food. Don't forget food. You can go a week without laughing."

—JOSS WHEDON

Enough talk—it's time to eat! Sure, it's one thing to understand how and why to be vegan (which are both great things), but it's something else entirely to get into the kitchen and get your hands dirty. Whipping up a delicious meal that satiates you, pleases your palate, and endears you to whomever you share it with is an experience second to none. You know what the best part is about vegan cooking? It's just like every other kind of cooking! Whether you're the kind of person who follows recipes with a stopwatch and always completely levels your teaspoons or you like to take an idea for something and then futz around with it to make it your own, these recipes will give you a great base repertoire to get started with. Breakfast, lunch, dinner, snacks, and desserts are all right here. You can spend all day creating a four-course feast (just saying, the Double Red Soup, Rainbow Vegetable Salad, Stovetop Mac and Cheese, and Fabulous Fudgy Brownies would make for an excellent dinner party), or just throw together a super-simple but totally satisfying meal like the Pasta and Greens Toss on a busy weeknight. Share these meals with people you love, adjust them to suit your tastes, and dig in to the wonderful, vast, and delicious world of vegan eating.

Breakfast

Tofu Scramble

Serves 4

For a hearty, savory breakfast, there's nothing like a tofu scramble. It's the perfect mixture of spices, vegetables, and filling tofu.

- **1 tablespoon extra-virgin olive oil**
- **½ cup chopped red onion**
- **½ red bell pepper, seeded and chopped**
- **1 cup sliced white mushrooms**
- **3 scallions, minced**
- **One 14-ounce package firm tofu, drained and crumbled**
- **¼ cup nutritional yeast (see Note)**
- **½ teaspoon smoked paprika**
- **½ teaspoon ground coriander**
- **½ teaspoon ground cumin**
- **¼ teaspoon ground turmeric**
- **Salt and freshly ground black pepper**

1. Heat the oil in a large skillet over medium heat. Add the onion and bell pepper and cook until softened, about 5 minutes. Add the mushrooms and scallions and cook until softened, about 4 minutes.
2. Stir in the tofu, nutritional yeast, paprika, coriander, cumin, turmeric, and salt and pepper to taste. Cook, stirring, until any remaining liquid has evaporated and the ingredients are hot, about 10 minutes. Serve hot.

* ***NOTE: Available in natural foods stores or online, nutritional yeast is a nonactive yeast—not to be confused with brewer's yeast or active dry yeast. Nutritional yeast provides a unique cheesy, umami flavor to foods and is a good source of vitamin B_{12}.***

Breakfast Burritos

Serves 4

Mornings sometimes need a little jolt to get you on your feet, and a delicious tofu scramble wrapped in a warm tortilla and topped with salsa is the perfect way to get going.

- **1 tablespoon extra-virgin olive oil**
- **1 large red onion, chopped**
- **1 yellow bell pepper, seeded and chopped**
- **4 ounces fresh mushrooms, chopped**
- **1 ripe tomato, chopped**
- **One 14-ounce package extra-firm tofu, drained and crumbled**
- **1 teaspoon ground cumin**
- **1 teaspoon ground coriander**
- **1 teaspoon salt**
- **¼ teaspoon freshly ground black pepper**
- **½ cup tomato salsa**
- **½ cup vegan sour cream**
- **4 large (8- to 10-inch) flour tortillas, warmed**

1. Heat the oil in a large skillet over medium-high heat. Add the onion and cook until softened, about 4 minutes. Add the bell pepper and mushrooms and cook until softened, about 5 minutes longer.
2. Stir in the tomato, tofu, cumin, coriander, salt, and pepper and cook, stirring, to heat through and blend the flavors, about 5 minutes. Continue cooking until any liquid has evaporated. Taste and adjust the seasonings if needed. Keep warm.
3. In a small bowl, combine the salsa and sour cream.
4. To serve, divide the tofu mixture among the tortillas, spooning it just below the center of each tortilla. Spoon ¼ cup of the salsa mixture onto the tofu mixture on each tortilla, then carefully roll up the tortillas. Serve hot.

Spinach-Tomato Frittata

Serves 4

If you thought eggy dishes like frittatas were off the menu without eggs, think again. Tofu is a great substitute for eggs. Use this recipe as a base and customize according to the seasons or your favorite veggies.

- **1 tablespoon extra-virgin olive oil**
- **1 medium yellow onion, chopped**
- **2 garlic cloves, chopped**
- **2 cups frozen chopped spinach, thawed**
- **1 teaspoon dried basil**
- **Salt and freshly ground black pepper**
- **One 14-ounce package firm tofu, drained and pressed (see Note)**
- **3 tablespoons nutritional yeast (see Note, page 152)**
- **1 tablespoon cornstarch**
- **1 tablespoon fresh lemon juice**
- **⅓ cup oil-packed or reconstituted sun-dried tomatoes, chopped**

1. Preheat the oven to 350°F. Lightly oil a deep 9- to 10-inch pie plate or a shallow baking dish and set aside.
2. Heat the oil in a skillet over medium-high heat. Add the onion and garlic and cook until softened, about 5 minutes.
3. Add the spinach and basil and cook until the spinach is tender and any liquid has evaporated, about 4 minutes. Season with salt and pepper to taste.
4. Transfer the spinach mixture to a food processor. Add the tofu, nutritional yeast, cornstarch, and lemon juice. Add salt and pepper to taste and process until smooth.

5. Scrape the mixture into the prepared pie plate. Mix in the sun-dried tomatoes and spread the mixture evenly, smoothing the top. Bake for about 45 minutes, until firm and golden brown. Serve hot.

* ***NOTE:** To press tofu, drain it well, wrap the tofu block in a clean kitchen towel, then place it in a rimmed baking pan and top with another baking pan or a cutting board, along with some canned goods to add weight. Set aside for about 30 minutes, then unwrap the tofu. It will be firmer and ready to use in recipes.*

Benedict Breakfast Stacks with Shortcut Hollandaise

Serves 4

Benedicts are some of mankind's all-time greatest creations. Making this for someone special on a lazy Saturday morning is a sure way to show you care.

- **12 ounces extra-firm tofu, drained and pressed (see Note, page 155)**
- **2 tablespoons all-purpose flour**
- **2 tablespoons nutritional yeast (see Note, page 152)**
- **½ teaspoon salt**
- **½ teaspoon freshly ground black pepper**
- **½ teaspoon smoked paprika**
- **Pinch of ground turmeric**
- **1 tablespoon neutral-flavored vegetable oil**
- **4 English muffins**
- **1 tablespoon vegan butter, such as Earth Balance**
- **1 large ripe tomato, cut into 8 thin slices**
- **8 to 16 slices Tempeh Bacon (page 158)**
- **Shortcut Hollandaise (recipe follows)**
- **2 tablespoons minced fresh scallions or chives**

1. Cut the tofu horizontally into 8 slabs.
2. In a shallow bowl, combine the flour, nutritional yeast, salt, pepper, paprika, and turmeric. Mix well. Dredge the tofu in the flour mixture and shake off any excess.
3. Heat the oil in a medium skillet over medium-high heat. Add the tofu slices and cook until golden brown on both sides, 5 to 7 minutes per side. Keep warm.
4. Toast the English muffins and spread with the vegan butter. Place two muffin halves on each serving plate, buttered side up. Top each half with a slice of tomato, followed by a slice of tofu and 1 or 2 bacon slices.

5. Spoon the hollandaise sauce on top of each stack, sprinkle with scallions, and serve immediately, allowing two stacks per person.

* ***NOTE: This recipe can easily be scaled up or down, depending on how many people you are serving. You can cook all of the tofu and bacon and then just reheat as much as you need at a time.***

Shortcut Hollandaise

Makes about 1 cup

Hollandaise is typically an emulsion of eggs, but this quick version boasts all the tangy richness of the original without any animal protein.

- **¾ cup vegan mayonnaise**
- **2 tablespoons fresh lemon juice**
- **1 tablespoon nutritional yeast (see Note, page 152)**
- **1½ teaspoons Dijon mustard**
- **⅛ teaspoon salt**
- **Pinch of cayenne**

1. Combine all the ingredients in a bowl or mini food processor or blender and blend until smooth.
2. Serve at once or transfer to a small bowl, cover tightly, and refrigerate until needed, up to 3 days. Serve at room temperature or warm gently when ready to use.

Tempeh Bacon

Serves 4

You'll need something to go alongside your scramble or hash, and tempeh bacon nails it. Not as crispy as pig-based bacon, tempeh bacon is all about the smoky seasoning.

- **One 8-ounce package tempeh**
- **3 tablespoons soy sauce**
- **3 tablespoons pure maple syrup**
- **1 tablespoon water**
- **1 teaspoon liquid smoke (see Note)**
- **½ teaspoon smoked paprika**
- **¼ teaspoon freshly ground black pepper**
- **¼ teaspoon garlic powder (optional)**
- **1 to 2 tablespoons extra-virgin olive oil**

1. Steam the tempeh in a steamer over simmering water for 15 minutes, then set aside to cool. Once cool, cut the tempeh into 12 to 14 very thin slices. Set aside.
2. In a shallow 8-inch baking dish, combine the soy sauce, maple syrup, water, and liquid smoke. Stir in the paprika, pepper, and garlic powder.
3. Add the tempeh strips to the marinade, turning to coat. Set aside for 30 minutes to marinate, or cover and refrigerate for several hours or overnight.
4. Heat the oil in a nonstick skillet over medium-high heat. Add the tempeh strips and cook until nicely browned and crisp on one side, 3 to 4 minutes. Flip the strips and cook the other side until crisp, about 3 minutes longer. Drizzle on the remaining marinade as the tempeh cooks, cooking for another minute or two, until the liquid is absorbed. Serve hot. Leftovers should be tightly covered and refrigerated for up to 5 days.

* ***NOTE: Available in small bottles in supermarkets, liquid smoke is a flavoring of concentrated smoky water that adds a grilled/smoked flavor to foods.***

Banana-Nut Muffins

Makes 12 muffins

Easy, filling, and sweet. Make a batch of these muffins on the weekend and you're set for a week's worth of breakfast.

- **2 large or 3 medium very ripe bananas, peeled and well mashed**
- **¾ cup natural sugar, such as Sugar in the Raw**
- **⅓ cup plain unsweetened nondairy milk, such as almond milk**
- **2 tablespoons neutral-flavored vegetable oil**
- **2 cups unbleached all-purpose flour or whole wheat pastry flour**
- **1 teaspoon baking soda**
- **½ teaspoon baking powder**
- **1 teaspoon salt**
- **1 teaspoon ground cinnamon**
- **¾ cup chopped walnuts or pecans**

1. Preheat the oven to 375°F. Lightly oil a 12-cup muffin pan and set aside.
2. In a large bowl, combine the bananas, sugar, nondairy milk, and oil and blend until smooth. Set aside.
3. In a separate bowl, combine the flour, baking soda, baking powder, salt, and cinnamon. Mix the dry ingredients into the wet ingredients just until blended. (Do not overmix or the muffins will be tough.)
4. Fold in the walnuts, then transfer the batter to the prepared pan, filling the cups about two-thirds full.
5. Bake for 25 minutes or until golden brown and a toothpick inserted in a muffin comes out clean. Set aside to cool. Once completely cool, the muffins can be stored tightly covered in the refrigerator for up to 1 week or frozen for up to 3 weeks.

Sweet Potato Hash

Serves 4

The homey deliciousness of sweet potatoes and savory seasonings makes hash a great addition to any brunch menu. For convenience, bake a few sweet potatoes in advance so you have them on hand. Otherwise you can peel and dice raw sweet potatoes and then steam or roast them until tender.

- **1 tablespoon extra-virgin olive oil**
- **1 large red onion, chopped**
- **1 small red or yellow bell pepper, seeded and chopped**
- **1 cup finely chopped mushrooms**
- **1 tablespoon soy sauce**
- **½ teaspoon dried thyme**
- **Salt and freshly ground black pepper**
- **1½ pounds sweet potatoes, cooked, peeled, and diced (about 3 cups)**
- **½ cup frozen green peas, thawed**

1. Heat the oil in a large skillet over medium-high heat. Add the onion and bell pepper and cook until softened, about 7 minutes.
2. Add the mushrooms, soy sauce, thyme, and salt and pepper to taste. Cook until softened, about 2 minutes, then add the sweet potatoes and peas. Cook, turning the mixture frequently, until the hash is hot and slightly browned, about 10 minutes. Serve hot.

Oatmeal as You Like It

Serves 4

Why settle for plain old oats when the combinations of additions and toppings are nearly endless? Mix and match from a variety of add-ins to wake up your taste buds and enjoy the classic bowl just the way you like it.

- **4 cups water**
- **2 cups old-fashioned rolled oats**
- **1 teaspoon ground cinnamon**
- **¼ teaspoon salt**

ADD-INS:

- **Raisins or sweetened dried cranberries**
- **Vegan granola**
- **Toasted slivered almonds or pecans**
- **Pure maple syrup, agave nectar, or fruit-sweetened jam**
- **Fresh fruit: sliced banana, ripe berries, chopped ripe peach**

1. Bring the water to a boil in a medium saucepan over high heat. Reduce the heat to medium-low and stir in the oats, cinnamon, and salt. Cover and simmer for 5 minutes, stirring occasionally.
2. Remove from the heat and let stand for 2 to 3 minutes.
3. Serve as you like it, stirring your choice of add-ins into the pot or spooning the unadorned oatmeal into serving bowls and passing the toppings in separate small bowls so everyone can customize his or her own serving.

Cinnamon-Raisin Pancakes

Serves 4

Not sure whether to make cinnamon rolls or pancakes? These flapjacks are a delicious, satisfying compromise.

- **1½ cups unbleached all-purpose flour**
- **¼ cup natural sugar, such as Sugar in the Raw**
- **1½ teaspoons ground cinnamon**
- **2 teaspoons baking powder**
- **½ teaspoon salt**
- **2 tablespoons ground flaxseeds**
- **¼ cup warm water**
- **1¼ cups almond milk**
- **1 teaspoon pure vanilla extract**
- **½ cup golden raisins**
- **Warm maple syrup for serving**

1. In a large bowl, combine the flour, sugar, cinnamon, baking powder, and salt. Set aside. In a blender, combine the flaxseeds and water and blend until thickened. Add the almond milk and vanilla and blend until smooth.
2. Pour the wet ingredients into the dry ingredients, mixing quickly until just moist. (Do not overmix or the pancakes will be tough.) Fold in the raisins.
3. Preheat the oven to 200°F. Heat a lightly oiled griddle or large non-stick skillet over medium heat.
4. Ladle about ¼ cup of the batter onto the hot griddle. Cook on one side until small bubbles appear on top, about 3 minutes. Flip the pancake with a metal spatula and cook until the other side is lightly browned, about 2 minutes longer.
5. Keep the cooked pancakes warm in the oven while you prepare the remaining pancakes. Serve hot with warm maple syrup.

Everyday Smoothie

Serves 1

Really, this smoothie is so simple and so satisfying you might make it every single day. Want to know a secret about smoothies? The key is to use frozen fruits (and vegetables!) so that you needn't add ice to get the thick, milk-shakey satisfaction that makes smoothies wonderful. If you use fresh fruit instead, add ½ cup ice to the blender for thickness.

- 1 frozen banana, cut into chunks, or 5 frozen strawberries
- ½ scoop chocolate protein powder, preferably Vega One
- 1½ cups coconut milk (see Note)
- ¼ cup frozen kale (see Note)

1. Combine all the ingredients in a blender and blend until smooth.
2. Pour into a large glass and serve.

* ***NOTES:** Know your coconut milks. The kind that comes in a carton (like dairy milk) is what you want to use with this recipe. The canned varieties are much thicker and are really good in curries, soups, and baking but are a bit too much for drinking straight.*

To freeze kale, simply remove and discard any tough stems, wash the kale well, and spin dry. Put the kale into resealable plastic bags and place in the freezer.

Lunch

Kale Salad

Serves 4

These days it's sacrilege to be a vegan and not have a favorite kale salad recipe. This one makes a great base that you can customize with add-ins as you like. I eat kale at least once a day—I think it's insanely good. Leftovers of this salad will keep in the refrigerator overnight, but after that the avocado will begin to turn brown.

- **1 bunch kale, washed, stemmed, and torn into bite-sized pieces**
- **1 Hass avocado, peeled, pitted, and chopped**
- **1 teaspoon rice wine vinegar**
- **1 teaspoon fresh lime juice**
- **½ teaspoon salt**

1. Combine all the ingredients in a large bowl.
2. Use your fingers to rub the avocado onto the kale leaves until the kale is well coated, then toss to combine. Allow the salad to sit for 5 minutes before serving.

* ***NOTE: To customize this recipe, add chopped scallions, grated carrots, a little stone-ground mustard, or artichoke hearts to the mix. Make it your own. The only must is the avocado.***

Rainbow Vegetable Salad

Serves 4

Here's a salad recipe without kale, but the abundance of colorful vegetables in this one pretty much makes up for it. This filling salad will keep for about four days in the fridge if you add the avocado later and only dress individual servings and leave the rest undressed until you're ready to eat it. It makes a great, easy lunch to pack for work.

- **One 15-ounce can chickpeas, drained and rinsed**
- **One 15-ounce can hearts of palm, drained and chopped**
- **1 head romaine lettuce, chopped**
- **1 red beet, peeled and grated**
- **1 golden beet, peeled and grated**
- **1 small fennel bulb, cored and thinly sliced**
- **1 large Hass avocado, peeled, pitted, and chopped**
- **Poppy seed salad dressing, such as Brianna's**

1. In a large bowl, combine the chickpeas, hearts of palm, lettuce, beets, and fennel.
2. If serving right away, add the avocado, pour on the dressing, and toss to combine. Otherwise, cover and refrigerate, then add the avocado and dressing when ready to serve.

Quinoa and Black Bean Salad

Serves 4

Quinoa is a nutritious staple full of fiber and protein, but on its own it can be a little bland. Mixing it with black beans, veggies, and a blend of seasonings makes it really stand out.

- **½ teaspoon salt, plus salt for cooking the quinoa**
- **1½ cups quinoa, thoroughly rinsed**
- **Two 15-ounce cans black beans, drained and rinsed**
- **1 ripe tomato, chopped**
- **1 cup cooked fresh or frozen corn kernels**
- **⅓ cup minced scallions**
- **¼ cup chopped fresh cilantro or parsley**
- **3 tablespoons extra-virgin olive oil**
- **2 tablespoons cider vinegar**
- **¼ teaspoon freshly ground black pepper**

1. Bring 3 cups of water to a boil in a saucepan. Add a pinch of salt. Add the quinoa, reduce the heat to low, cover, and simmer for 15 to 20 minutes, or until the water is absorbed and the quinoa is tender. Drain any remaining water and blot the quinoa to remove excess moisture.
2. Place the cooked quinoa in a serving bowl. Add the black beans, tomato, corn, scallions, and cilantro.
3. In a small bowl, combine the olive oil, vinegar, ½ teaspoon salt, and pepper. Pour the dressing over the salad and toss well to combine.
4. Cover and set aside for 15 minutes before serving or cover tightly and refrigerate until ready to serve. Properly stored, the salad will keep in the refrigerator for up to 3 days.

Noodle Salad with Peanut Sauce

Serves 4

This might be called a salad, but it's really a meal all on its own. Chock-full of colorful vegetables, rice noodles, tofu, and a slightly spicy peanut sauce, it's as filling as any entrée.

FOR THE SALAD

- **One 8-ounce package rice noodles**
- **1 red bell pepper, seeded and sliced**
- **1 yellow bell pepper, seeded and sliced**
- **4 cups shredded red and green cabbage**
- **1 bunch fresh basil, chopped**
- **4 scallions, chopped**

FOR THE PEANUT SAUCE

- **1 cup peanut butter**
- **½ cup soy sauce**
- **2 garlic cloves, crushed**
- **One 2-inch piece fresh ginger, peeled and sliced**
- **¼ cup rice wine vinegar**
- **½ cup water**

1. Cook the rice noodles according to the package directions. Drain well, then transfer to a large bowl.
2. Add the bell peppers, cabbage, basil, and scallions to the bowl.
3. In a blender or food processor, combine the peanut butter, soy sauce, garlic, ginger, vinegar, and water. Blend until smooth, about 2 minutes.
4. Pour the sauce over the noodle mixture and toss to coat. Serve immediately or cover and refrigerate until needed. Leftovers will keep in the refrigerator for up to 4 days.

Garden Wraps with Hummus

Serves 4

Maybe it's a vegan stereotype to love hummus, but simple, veggie-filled wraps like these are the reason for the admiration.

- **1 cup Here's My Hummus (page 195) or purchased hummus**
- **¼ cup minced red onion**
- **¼ cup sliced, pitted Kalamata olives**
- **¼ cup chopped reconstituted or oil-packed sun-dried tomatoes**
- **2 tablespoons minced fresh parsley or basil**
- **4 large (8- to 10-inch) flour tortillas or lavash flatbread**
- **2 cups shredded romaine lettuce**
- **1 large carrot, grated**
- **2 ripe tomatoes, thinly sliced**
- **1 English cucumber, peeled and cut into ¼-inch strips**
- **1 ripe Hass avocado, peeled, pitted, and sliced**
- **Salt and freshly ground black pepper**
- **Hot sauce (optional)**

1. In a bowl, combine the hummus, onion, olives, sun-dried tomatoes, and parsley, stirring to mix well. Set aside.
2. To assemble the wraps, divide the hummus mixture among the tortillas and spread evenly across the surface.
3. Spread the lettuce and carrot over the hummus, then arrange a few slices of tomato, cucumber, and avocado across the bottom half of each tortilla. Season to taste with salt, pepper, and hot sauce.
4. Roll up the wraps tightly, then slice in half diagonally. Serve immediately.

Easy Bean and Rice Burritos

Serves 4

If you don't happen to live in a town with great Mexican food, step one is to visit San Francisco. Step two is to make these hearty bean-filled burritos at home.

- **1 tablespoon extra-virgin olive oil**
- **1 yellow onion, chopped**
- **1 red bell pepper, seeded and chopped**
- **One 15-ounce can pinto, black, or red kidney beans, drained and rinsed**
- **1 cup tomato salsa**
- **1 cup cooked brown rice**
- **4 large (8- to 10-inch) flour tortillas**
- **½ cup shredded vegan cheese (optional)**
- **1 Hass avocado, peeled, pitted, and thinly sliced**
- **Hot sauce (optional)**

1. Heat the oil in a saucepan over medium heat. Add the onion and bell pepper, cover, and cook until softened, about 5 minutes.

2. Add the beans and salsa and cook, mashing the beans and stirring to combine. Cook for a few minutes to heat through.

3. If needed, heat the rice in a microwave or in a small saucepan.

4. To warm the tortillas, wrap them in foil and place them in a 275°F oven for a few minutes.

5. To serve, spoon about ½ cup of the bean mixture down the center of each tortilla. Top with the rice, followed by the cheese. Top with avocado slices and hot sauce to taste. Roll up the burritos, tucking in the sides, and serve hot.

Vegetable Fajitas

Serves 4

Sizzling right from the stovetop, fajitas are a great option when you're serving both vegans and omnivores. No one can resist seared bell peppers and onions with authentic spices and slices of fresh avocado.

- **1 tablespoon extra-virgin olive oil**
- **1 large red onion, halved lengthwise and cut into strips**
- **1 large bell pepper (any color), seeded and cut lengthwise into ¼-inch strips**
- **2 large portobello mushroom caps, cut into ¼-inch strips**
- **1 medium zucchini, trimmed and cut into ¼-inch strips**
- **½ teaspoon ground cumin**
- **½ teaspoon dried oregano**
- **Salt and freshly ground black pepper**
- **4 large (8- to 10-inch) flour tortillas**
- **1 cup tomato salsa**
- **1 ripe Hass avocado, peeled, pitted, and thinly sliced**

1. Heat the oil in a large skillet over medium-high heat. Add the onion and bell pepper and cook, stirring, until seared on the outside, about 4 minutes.

2. Add the mushrooms and zucchini. Season with the cumin, the oregano, and salt and pepper to taste. Cook, stirring occasionally, until all the vegetables are tender, about 5 minutes longer.

3. To warm the tortillas, wrap them in foil and place them in a 275°F oven for a few minutes.

4. To assemble, spoon the vegetable mixture onto each of the tortillas, just below the center, dividing evenly. Spoon some salsa onto the vegetables and top each with avocado slices. Roll up the tortillas to enclose the filling. Serve immediately.

Curried Tofu Salad Pitas

Serves 4

If stuffing a soft pita full of delicious curried tofu salad (think chicken salad, minus our fowl friends) is wrong, who wants to be right? I like to make this salad at least half an hour ahead of time, or even the day before, to allow the flavors to meld.

- **¼ cup plain coconut milk yogurt**
- **¼ cup vegan mayonnaise**
- **1½ teaspoons curry powder, or more to taste**
- **½ teaspoon salt, or more to taste**
- **One 14-ounce package extra-firm tofu, drained and patted dry**
- **1 celery rib, minced**
- **4 scallions, minced**
- **¼ cup raisins**
- **¼ cup chopped dry-roasted cashews**
- **¼ cup finely chopped mango or apple**
- **4 whole-grain pitas, halved**
- **Lettuce leaves or alfalfa sprouts for serving**

1. In a large bowl, combine the yogurt, mayonnaise, curry powder, and salt. Stir to mix well, then taste and adjust the seasonings, adding more curry powder or salt if desired. Set aside.
2. Cut the tofu into ½-inch dice and add to the curry sauce. Add the celery, scallions, raisins, cashews, and mango. Stir to combine thoroughly.
3. Cover and refrigerate for 30 minutes to allow the flavors to develop. Taste and adjust the seasonings if needed.
4. To serve, spoon the tofu mixture inside each of the pita halves along with a lettuce leaf or alfalfa sprouts.

Chickpea Salad Sandwiches

Serves 4

Layered with lettuce and tomato, this salad makes an easy, satisfying alternative to those tired old egg salad and tuna salad sandwiches.

- **One 15-ounce can chickpeas, drained and rinsed**
- **½ cup chopped celery**
- **2 scallions, minced**
- **2 tablespoons minced red onion**
- **½ cup vegan mayonnaise, or more if needed**
- **2 teaspoons Dijon mustard**
- **2 teaspoons fresh lemon juice**
- **1 teaspoon capers, chopped**
- **2 teaspoons minced fresh dill (optional)**
- **Salt and freshly ground black pepper**
- **Bread of choice, toasted**
- **Lettuce leaves and sliced ripe tomato for serving**

1. Place the chickpeas in a bowl and mash them. Add the celery, scallions, onion, mayonnaise, mustard, lemon juice, capers, and dill. Season to taste with salt and pepper, then mix well to combine. Taste and adjust the seasonings if needed. Add a little more mayo if the mixture is too dry. For the best flavor, cover and refrigerate for 30 minutes to allow the flavors to blend.

2. Scoop the chickpea salad onto your choice of toasted bread and top with lettuce and tomato to make each sandwich. Alternatively, you can serve the chickpea salad in lettuce leaves or make it into open-face sandwiches by topping single slices of bread with the chickpea salad as for bruschette. Leftover chickpea salad can be stored in the refrigerator in a tightly covered container for up to 3 days.

Sloppy Janes

Serves 4

Toothsome and flavorful, shiitake mushrooms transform into limitless meat stand-ins. These yummy burgers are perfect with a side of Fritos (yes, Fritos are vegan!).

- **1 tablespoon extra-virgin olive oil**
- **1 yellow onion, chopped**
- **1 green bell pepper, seeded and chopped**
- **3 garlic cloves, minced**
- **12 ounces fresh shiitake mushrooms, stemmed and chopped**
- **One 15-ounce can pinto beans, drained, rinsed, and mashed**
- **1 cup ketchup**
- **2 tablespoons tomato paste**
- **1 tablespoon red wine vinegar**
- **1 tablespoon molasses**
- **1 tablespoon vegan Worcestershire sauce or soy sauce**
- **1 tablespoon Dijon mustard**
- **2 teaspoons natural sugar, such as Sugar in the Raw**
- **1 teaspoon chili powder**
- **¼ teaspoon cayenne (optional)**
- **Salt and freshly ground black pepper**
- **4 sandwich rolls, split**

1. Heat the oil in a large skillet over medium heat. Add the onion and bell pepper and cook until softened, about 5 minutes. Stir in the garlic and cook for 1 minute longer, then add the mushrooms and cook, stirring, until tender, about 4 minutes.

2. Stir in the mashed pinto beans, ketchup, tomato paste, vinegar, and molasses. Add the Worcestershire sauce, mustard, sugar, chili powder, cayenne, and salt and pepper to taste. Simmer for 10 minutes, stirring. Adjust the seasonings. Add a little water if the mixture becomes dry.

3. Spoon the shiitake mixture onto split rolls and serve hot. If you have any leftover shiitake mixture, it will keep well in the refrigerator in a tightly covered container for up to 3 days.

Dinner

Soyrizo Pasta

Serves 4

Hearty, homey, and boasting a tiny kick, this pasta couldn't be easier. You'd never guess that it has only five ingredients—it's just as delicious as it is quick to prepare, which makes it a go-to for weeknight dinners when you're short on time. A little bit of spice from the Soyrizo perks up the tangy tomatoes.

- **One 16-ounce box farfalle, penne, or other bite-sized pasta**
- **Salt**
- **2 teaspoons extra-virgin olive oil**
- **3 garlic cloves, chopped**
- **One 28-ounce can crushed tomatoes**
- **One 12-ounce package Soyrizo**

1. Cook the pasta in a pot of boiling salted water according to the package directions. Drain well and set aside.
2. Heat the oil in a large skillet over medium heat. Add the garlic and cook for 2 minutes.
3. Add the tomatoes and Soyrizo, reduce the heat to medium-low, and cook for 10 more minutes, stirring occasionally.
4. Add the cooked pasta and toss to coat, stirring to heat through for about 2 minutes. Serve warm. Leftovers will keep, covered, for up to 5 days in the fridge.

Black Bean Burgers

Serves 4

What would the weekly menu be without burger night? These burgers can be made ahead and then wrapped individually and frozen for future use.

- **½ cup old-fashioned rolled oats, or more as needed**
- **½ cup walnut pieces**
- **¼ cup minced scallion**
- **2 tablespoons minced fresh parsley**
- **One 15-ounce can black beans, drained, rinsed, and blotted dry**
- **2 teaspoons cornstarch or tapioca starch, or more as needed**
- **½ teaspoon garlic powder**
- **½ teaspoon smoked paprika**
- **½ teaspoon dried basil, dried thyme, or ground cumin (optional)**
- **Salt and freshly ground black pepper**
- **2 tablespoons extra-virgin olive oil**
- **4 burger buns, split**
- **Choice of accompaniments: lettuce leaves, sliced tomato, avocado, or onion; relish, pickle slices, ketchup, mustard, or vegan mayonnaise**

1. In a food processor, combine the oats and walnuts and grind finely. Add the scallion, parsley, beans, cornstarch, garlic powder, paprika, basil, and salt and pepper to taste. Process until well combined, leaving some texture.

2. Pinch the mixture with your fingers to see if it holds together. If the mixture is too dry, add a teaspoon or two of water and mix again. If the mixture is too wet, add more oats or cornstarch. Shape the mixture into 4 burgers and refrigerate for 30 minutes.

3. Heat the oil in a large nonstick skillet over medium heat. Add the burgers and cook until browned on both sides, turning once, about 5 minutes per side.

4. Serve the burgers on the buns, with your choice of toppings.

Double Red Soup

Serves 4

Red lentils and roasted red peppers were made for each other. The peppers give hearty lentils a little tanginess. This easy, warming soup is especially good with rustic bread (like a bâtard or an olive loaf). Serve with a side of Kale Salad (page 165) to make a satisfying dinner.

- **2 tablespoons extra-virgin olive oil**
- **1 large yellow onion, chopped**
- **4 garlic cloves, chopped**
- **4 roasted red peppers, fresh (see Note) or from a jar, chopped**
- **6 cups water**
- **2 tablespoons vegan bouillon paste, such as Better than Bouillon (see Note)**
- **One 28-ounce can whole or diced tomatoes, undrained**
- **2 cups dried whole red lentils, any stones removed**
- **2 teaspoons rice wine vinegar**
- **Salt and freshly ground black pepper**

1. Heat the oil in a large pot over medium-high heat. Add the onion and cook until nearly translucent, about 3 minutes. Add the garlic and peppers and cook for 2 minutes longer.

2. Stir in the water, bouillon, tomatoes, and lentils and bring to a boil. Boil for 3 minutes, then reduce the heat to medium and simmer, uncovered, until the lentils are tender and begin to split open, 10 to 15 minutes. Remove from the heat.

3. Using an immersion blender or a regular blender, blend the soup until smooth. Add the vinegar, then taste and add salt and pepper to taste. Serve warm. Store leftovers in a tightly covered container in the refrigerator for up to 5 days or in the freezer for 3 to 4 weeks.

* *NOTES: Roast your own peppers by halving them and placing them under a broiler cut side down for 10 minutes, until the skins are completely blackened. Turn them after a few minutes so all sides brown. Let the peppers cool in a covered bowl or in a paper bag. Then carefully remove the skins, and they're ready to eat or cook.*

Available in supermarkets and online, Better than Bouillon Vegetarian Bases are highly concentrated pastes that make a rich broth when combined with water.

Pasta and Greens Toss

Serves 4

I love grain bowls (meals that involve a cooked grain, greens, protein, and sauce, all served in a bowl), but this version cuts down on cooking time by replacing rice with pasta. More of a technique than a recipe, this dish is endlessly customizable. Choose your favorite green vegetable and toss it with your preferred pasta and a touch of garlic and capers.

- **One 16-ounce box farfalle or other bite-sized pasta**
- **Salt**
- **¼ cup extra-virgin olive oil**
- **4 garlic cloves, minced**
- **2 teaspoons capers**
- **2 cups broccoli florets, fresh or frozen**
- **2 cups kale, washed, tough stems removed, torn into bite-sized pieces**
- **Salt and freshly ground black pepper**

1. Cook the pasta in a large pot of boiling salted water according to the package directions.
2. While the pasta is cooking, heat the oil in a small saucepan or skillet over medium heat. Add the garlic and cook, stirring, until softened, about 2 minutes. Remove from the heat before the garlic begins to brown. Stir in the capers and set aside.
3. Just before the pasta is done, add the broccoli to the pasta pot and cook for 2 minutes.
4. Place a large colander in the sink and put the kale in the colander. Pour the cooked pasta and broccoli over the kale and drain.
5. Return the saucepan to low heat for 1 or 2 minutes to warm the garlic-caper oil.
6. In a large serving bowl, combine the pasta, veggies, and garlic-caper oil. Season with salt and pepper to taste and toss gently to combine. Store leftovers in a tightly sealed container in the refrigerator for up to 3 days.

Tamari-Lemon Baked Tofu

Serves 4

Whether it's at the center of a grain bowl or served alongside steamed bok choy, perfectly seasoned tofu like this makes any meal complete.

- **One 14-ounce package extra-firm tofu, drained and blotted dry**
- **¼ cup tamari**
- **¼ cup water**
- **3 tablespoons fresh lemon juice**
- **2 tablespoons agave nectar**
- **1 tablespoon dark sesame oil**

1. Cut the tofu into ½-inch-thick slices. Place the slices on a baking sheet lined with paper towels. Cover with more paper towels and place another baking sheet on top along with some canned goods to press the liquid out of the tofu. Let it sit for 20 minutes.
2. In a small bowl, combine the tamari, water, lemon juice, agave nectar, and sesame oil. Blend well. Place the pressed tofu slices in a 9-by-13-inch glass baking dish and pour the marinade on top. Cover and refrigerate for 2 to 3 hours or overnight, turning the tofu once.
3. Preheat the oven to 375°F. Remove the tofu from the marinade and place on a lightly oiled baking sheet. Bake, drizzling on any remaining marinade, for about 45 minutes, until the tofu is browned and firm, turning once about halfway through the baking time. Serve hot. Leftovers can be stored in the refrigerator in a tightly sealed container for up to 3 days.

Kale and White Bean Soup

Serves 4

Soup is the amazingly versatile base for so many weekly menus. Cook up a pot of this rustic kale and white bean version and enjoy it throughout the week as the flavors continue to meld.

- **1 tablespoon extra-virgin olive oil**
- **1 large yellow onion, finely chopped**
- **3 to 4 garlic cloves, minced**
- **2 or 3 Yukon Gold potatoes, peeled and cut into ½-inch dice**
- **One 14.5-ounce can diced fire-roasted tomatoes**
- **Two 15-ounce cans cannellini or other white beans, drained and rinsed**
- **1 teaspoon dried oregano**
- **½ teaspoon smoked paprika**
- **¼ teaspoon red pepper flakes**
- **5 cups vegetable broth**
- **Salt and freshly ground black pepper**
- **9 ounces kale, any variety, coarsely chopped**

1. Heat the oil in a soup pot over medium heat. Add the onion, cover, and cook until softened, stirring occasionally, about 5 minutes. Remove the lid, add the garlic, and cook for 1 minute longer.

2. Stir in the potatoes, then add the tomatoes and their juice, white beans, oregano, paprika, red pepper flakes, and vegetable broth. Season with salt and pepper to taste. Bring to a boil, then reduce the heat to medium and simmer for 15 minutes.

3. Stir in the kale and cook for another 10 minutes or until the vegetables are tender. Taste and adjust the seasonings if needed. Serve hot. Store leftovers in a tightly sealed container in the refrigerator for up to 5 days or in the freezer for 3 to 4 weeks.

Pasta with Artichoke Alfredo

Serves 4

Think that cream sauces are verboten for vegans? Not so fast. Once you master the technique here, you can riff off the base recipe for any dish that calls for a savory cream sauce.

- **3 garlic cloves, crushed**
- **One 12-ounce jar (or two 6-ounce jars) marinated artichoke hearts, drained**
- **One 15-ounce can cannellini or other white beans, drained and rinsed**
- **½ cup vegetable broth**
- **½ cup plain unsweetened almond milk**
- **2 tablespoons nutritional yeast (see Note, page 152)**
- **2 tablespoons fresh lemon juice**
- **1 teaspoon dried basil**
- **Salt and freshly ground black pepper**
- **One 12-ounce box dried pasta of your choice**
- **2 tablespoons minced fresh Italian parsley**

1. Finely mince the garlic in a food processor or blender (see Note). Add the artichoke hearts, white beans, and vegetable broth and process until smooth. Add the almond milk, nutritional yeast, lemon juice, basil, and salt and pepper to taste. Process until smooth. Taste and adjust the seasonings if needed. Set aside.

2. Cook the pasta in boiling salted water according to the package directions. Drain well and return to the pot.

3. Add the sauce to the pasta and toss gently to combine and heat through. Serve hot sprinkled with the parsley. Store leftovers in the refrigerator in a tightly covered container for up to 5 days.

* ***NOTE: For a truly creamy sauce, using a Vitamix or other high-speed blender works best. These machines are no joke—they can blend*** **anything.**

Portobello and Cremini Stroganoff

Serves 4

This paprika-infused delight traditionally made with beef is just as rich and hearty as the original, thanks to the toothsome mushrooms. Vegan Worcestershire sauce adds extra depth and savoriness.

- **2 tablespoons tomato paste**
- **1 tablespoon vegan Worcestershire sauce or soy sauce**
- **1½ cups vegetable broth**
- **1 tablespoon extra-virgin olive oil**
- **2 yellow onions, chopped**
- **4 portobello mushrooms, trimmed, gills scraped, and cut into ¾-inch dice**
- **8 ounces cremini mushrooms, trimmed, halved, and sliced**
- **2 tablespoons unbleached all-purpose flour**
- **1 tablespoon sweet Hungarian paprika**
- **2 teaspoons smoked paprika**
- **Salt and freshly ground black pepper**
- **½ cup vegan sour cream**
- **Freshly cooked noodles for serving**

1. In a small bowl, combine the tomato paste and Worcestershire sauce with ¼ cup of the broth, blending until smooth. Set aside.

2. Heat the oil in a large, deep skillet or saucepan over medium-high heat. Add the onions, cover, and cook until softened, about 5 minutes. Uncover, add both kinds of mushrooms, and cook, stirring occasionally, until lightly browned all over, about 5 minutes.

3. Stir in the flour and both kinds of paprika. Cook, stirring, for about 1 minute, then add the tomato paste mixture, stirring until smooth.

4. Add the remaining 1¼ cups broth and bring to a boil. Reduce the heat to low and season with salt and pepper to taste. Simmer until the flavors are blended and the sauce thickens a little, about 25 minutes. Just before serving, slowly stir in the sour cream until well blended. Serve hot over noodles. Store leftovers in a tightly covered container in the refrigerator for up to 3 days.

Rice with Beans and Greens

Serves 4

It doesn't get more straightforward than a plate covered with a beautiful combination of rice, beans, and greens. These three staples are made to go together; whether or not you douse them in hot sauce is up to you.

- **1 tablespoon extra-virgin olive oil**
- **1 yellow onion, chopped**
- **3 garlic cloves, minced**
- **1 cup long-grain brown rice**
- **2 cups vegetable broth**
- **Salt and freshly ground black pepper**
- **9 ounces baby kale, spinach, or chard, coarsely chopped**
- **One 15-ounce can cannellini beans, chickpeas, or black beans, drained and rinsed**
- **2 tablespoons minced fresh parsley, basil, or cilantro**
- **1 tablespoon fresh lemon juice (optional)**
- **Choice of add-ins: chopped ripe tomato, chopped sun-dried tomatoes, pitted Kalamata olives, toasted pine nuts, raisins, hot sauce**

1. Heat the oil in a large, deep skillet or Dutch oven over medium heat. Add the onion and cook for 5 minutes or until softened. Add the garlic and cook for 1 minute longer.

2. Stir in the rice, then add the broth and salt and pepper to taste. (The amount of salt needed will depend on the saltiness of your broth.) Bring to a boil. Reduce the heat to low, cover, and simmer for 35 minutes or until the rice is almost tender.

3. Stir in the kale, then add the beans and continue cooking until the rice and vegetables are tender and all the liquid has been absorbed, 5 to 10 minutes longer.

4. Stir in the parsley and lemon juice and your choice of add-ins. Serve hot. Store leftovers in a tightly sealed container in the refrigerator for up to 5 days.

Black and Red Bean Chili

Serves 4

Dollop this spicy chili with vegan sour cream, garnish with scallions, and serve with your favorite corn bread or biscuits. If you prefer less heat, leave out the chipotle chile and use a mild chili powder.

- **1 tablespoon extra-virgin olive oil**
- **1 large onion, chopped**
- **1 carrot, chopped**
- **1 red or green bell pepper, seeded and chopped**
- **3 garlic cloves, minced**
- **2 tablespoons tomato paste**
- **1 chipotle chile in adobo sauce, minced**
- **2 tablespoons chili powder**
- **1 teaspoon ground cumin**
- **One 14.5-ounce can fire-roasted diced tomatoes, undrained**
- **One 15-ounce can black beans, drained and rinsed**
- **One 15-ounce can dark red kidney beans, drained and rinsed**
- **½ teaspoon salt**
- **¼ teaspoon freshly ground black pepper**
- **¾ cup water, or more as needed**
- **Choice of toppings: vegan sour cream, diced avocado, sliced black olives, chopped scallions**

1. Heat the oil in a large pot over medium heat. Add the onion, carrot, bell pepper, and garlic. Cover and cook until softened, about 5 minutes. Uncover and stir in the tomato paste and chipotle chile. Then stir in the chili powder, cumin, tomatoes, black beans, kidney beans, salt, and pepper.

2. Add the water and bring to a boil, then reduce the heat to low and simmer for 30 minutes or until the vegetables are tender and the flavors are blended. If you prefer a soupier texture, add more water. If you prefer the chili thicker, turn up the heat for a few minutes to evaporate some of the liquid. Taste and adjust the seasonings if needed.
3. Serve hot with your choice of toppings. Store leftovers in a tightly covered container in the refrigerator for up to 5 days or in the freezer for 3 to 4 weeks.

Stovetop Mac and Cheese

Serves 4

This mac and cheese has all the satisfying saltiness of the boxed original, but it is made from scratch. Whip this up for your friends and show them how your tastes have matured since college.

- **8 ounces elbow macaroni or other bite-sized pasta**
- **1 teaspoon salt, plus salt for cooking the macaroni**
- **¼ cup roasted red bell pepper (see Note, page 179) or solid-pack pumpkin puree**
- **2 tablespoons fresh lemon juice**
- **1 tablespoon tahini or almond butter**
- **1 teaspoon Dijon mustard**
- **¾ cup nutritional yeast (see Note, page 152)**
- **2 tablespoons cornstarch**
- **1 teaspoon onion powder**
- **½ teaspoon garlic powder**
- **½ teaspoon smoked paprika**
- **¼ teaspoon freshly ground black pepper**
- **2 cups plain unsweetened almond milk**
- **1 cup shredded vegan Cheddar cheese**

1. Cook the macaroni in a pot of boiling salted water until it is al dente. Drain and return to the pot. While the macaroni is cooking, combine the roasted red pepper, lemon juice, tahini, mustard, and nutritional yeast in a food processor or blender. Add the cornstarch, 1 teaspoon salt, the onion powder, garlic powder, paprika, and pepper. Add the almond milk and blend until completely smooth and creamy.

2. Add the sauce mixture to the pot containing the cooked and drained macaroni and cook, stirring, over medium heat until the sauce begins to thicken. Mix in the shredded cheese, stirring gently to melt. Taste and adjust the seasonings if needed. If the mixture becomes too thick, stir in a little extra almond milk or some vegetable broth. Serve hot. Store leftovers in a tightly sealed container in the refrigerator for up to 5 days.

Vegetable Fried Rice

Serves 4

A clever time-saver is to cook a big batch of rice during the weekend and then use it in meals throughout the week. Fried rice is the traditional way to use leftover rice, and it couldn't be more delicious.

- **1 cup extra-firm tofu, drained and pressed (see Note, page 155)**
- **3 tablespoons soy sauce, or more as needed**
- **Salt and freshly ground black pepper**
- **1 tablespoon neutral-flavored vegetable oil**
- **1 large yellow onion, chopped**
- **1 carrot, grated**
- **2 garlic cloves, minced**
- **3 scallions, minced**
- **1 teaspoon fresh ginger, peeled and grated**
- **3 cups cold cooked rice**
- **½ cup frozen green peas, thawed**
- **1 teaspoon dark sesame oil**

1. Crumble the tofu into a bowl. Add 1 tablespoon of the soy sauce, season with salt and pepper, and mix well. Set aside.

2. Heat the vegetable oil in a large skillet or wok over medium-high heat. Add the onion and carrot and stir-fry for 4 minutes. Add the garlic, scallions, and ginger and stir-fry for 30 seconds.

3. Add the rice, peas, sesame oil, and remaining 2 tablespoons soy sauce. Stir-fry to mix well, then stir in the reserved tofu mixture and stir-fry for 3 minutes longer to heat through. Taste and adjust the seasonings, adding more soy sauce or salt if needed. Store leftovers in a tightly sealed container in the refrigerator for up to 5 days.

Asian Noodle Stir-Fry

Serves 4

It's almost impossible to eat a vegan diet for an extended period of time without developing a favorite stir-fry recipe. Chewy noodles, crunchy vegetables, and a savory sauce make this dish a must-try.

- **¼ cup soy sauce**
- **¼ cup hoisin sauce**
- **2 tablespoons tahini or peanut butter**
- **2 teaspoons rice vinegar**
- **1 teaspoon Sriracha or Asian chili paste**
- **⅓ cup water**
- **8 ounces rice noodles or linguine**
- **2 teaspoons dark sesame oil**
- **1 tablespoon neutral-flavored vegetable oil**
- **1 carrot, grated or thinly sliced on the diagonal**
- **1 red bell pepper, seeded and cut into thin strips**
- **5 scallions, minced**
- **2 garlic cloves, minced**
- **2 teaspoons fresh ginger, peeled and minced**
- **8 ounces extra-firm tofu, drained, blotted dry, and cut into ½-inch dice**
- **2 ounces snow peas, trimmed and cut into 1-inch pieces**

1. In a small bowl, combine the soy sauce, hoisin sauce, tahini, vinegar, Sriracha, and water. Mix to combine well. Set aside.

2. Cook the noodles according to the package directions. Drain the noodles and return to the pot. Add the sesame oil and toss to coat.

3. Heat the vegetable oil in a large skillet or wok over medium-high heat. Add the carrot, bell pepper, scallions, garlic, and ginger and stir-fry until fragrant, about 30 seconds. Add the tofu and snow peas and stir-fry for 3 minutes. Add half of the reserved sauce and stir-fry to coat. Add the reserved noodles to the skillet along with the remaining sauce. Toss gently to combine and heat through. Serve hot. Store leftovers in a tightly sealed container in the refrigerator for up to 5 days.

Snacks and Sides

Sweet Potato Fries

Serves 4

There are two amazing things about sweet potato fries: they are fries, but through the magic of beta-carotene (and the fact that they're baked, not fried), they're also good for you. Like, whoa. Serve these alongside your favorite burgers or wraps.

- **1½ pounds sweet potatoes**
- **Extra-virgin olive oil**
- **Salt and freshly ground black pepper**

1. Preheat the oven to 425°F. Peel the sweet potatoes and cut them in half lengthwise. Place one cut half on a work surface and cut into ¼-inch slices. Repeat with the remaining potatoes. Transfer to a large bowl and drizzle on 1 to 2 tablespoons of olive oil. Season with salt and pepper and toss to coat.
2. Spread the sweet potatoes in a single layer on an oiled rimmed baking sheet and bake for 30 minutes or until the potatoes are tender and lightly browned, turning once about halfway through.
3. To serve, transfer the sweet potatoes to a bowl and sprinkle with a few grinds of black pepper and a little more salt if desired. Serve hot.

So-Good Guacamole

Serves 4

Avocados make everything better, but they are central to guacamole. Beyond the chip bowl, try this dolloped on your Sweet Potato Hash (page 160) or Tofu Scramble (page 152). And be sure to eat it all—guacamole is best the day it is made.

- **2 to 3 ripe Hass avocados**
- **1 tablespoon fresh lime juice**
- **¼ teaspoon salt**
- **¼ cup minced red onion or scallion**
- **2 tablespoons minced fresh cilantro**
- **1 jalapeño or serrano chile, seeded and minced (optional)**
- **1 garlic clove, minced (optional)**
- **1 plum tomato, finely chopped (optional)**
- **Tortilla chips for serving**

1. Halve and pit the avocados and scoop the flesh into a bowl.
2. Add the lime juice and salt and mash well. Add the onion, cilantro, jalapeño, garlic, and tomato. Mix well to combine.
3. Taste and adjust the seasonings, adding more salt or lime juice if needed. Serve with tortilla chips.

Roasted Chickpeas

Serves 4

Whether you like them savory, sweet, or spicy, roasted chickpeas are a versatile treat. Add these crunchy bites to your favorite salad or enjoy them on their own as a handy snack.

- **One 15-ounce can chickpeas, drained, rinsed, and blotted dry**
- **2 tablespoons extra-virgin olive oil**
- **Salt**
- **2 teaspoons garam masala or other spice blend (optional)**

1. Preheat the oven to 400°F. Lightly oil a shallow baking dish or a rimmed baking sheet (large enough to fit the chickpeas in a single layer) or spray it with cooking spray.
2. Spread the chickpeas in a single layer in the prepared baking pan and drizzle on the olive oil. Toss gently to coat. Season with salt to taste.
3. Roast the chickpeas, stirring occasionally, for about 30 minutes, until they begin to turn brown and crispy. Remove from the oven and sprinkle on the garam masala and a little more salt if needed. Allow to cool to room temperature. Store leftovers in a tightly sealed container in a cool, dry place for 3 to 5 days.

Here's My Hummus

Makes about 2 cups

Whether you dip vegetables into it, slather it liberally on sandwiches for extra heartiness, or use it as a base for more complex dips, there's no wrong way to indulge in hummus.

- **One 15-ounce can chickpeas, drained and rinsed**
- **2 garlic cloves, crushed**
- **¼ cup tahini**
- **3 tablespoons fresh lemon juice**
- **½ teaspoon salt**
- **¼ teaspoon smoked paprika or 1 tablespoon minced fresh parsley**
- **Pita chips or cut-up raw vegetables for serving**

1. In a food processor, combine the chickpeas and garlic and process to a paste. Add the tahini, lemon juice, and salt and process until smooth and completely blended.
2. Scrape the hummus into a bowl. Cover and refrigerate for 1 hour to allow the flavors to develop. Serve chilled or at room temperature, sprinkled with the paprika or parsley and accompanied by pita chips or vegetables for dipping. Store leftovers in a tightly sealed container in the refrigerator for up to 5 days.

Cheesy Kale Chips

Serves 4

There's nothing not to love about kale chips—but you can spend a fortune on the packaged kind. To enjoy the crunchy, cheesy treats without bankrupting your retirement fund, try this at-home version.

- **1 bunch curly kale, tough stems removed (see Note)**
- **¾ cup raw cashews, soaked in water for 3 or 4 hours and drained**
- **1 garlic clove, crushed**
- **½ cup nutritional yeast (see Note, page 152)**
- **2 tablespoons fresh lemon juice**
- **1 tablespoon soy sauce**
- **1 teaspoon prepared yellow mustard**
- **¼ teaspoon sea salt**
- **Water, as needed**

1. Tear or cut the kale leaves into 2-inch pieces and transfer to a large bowl. Set aside.
2. Preheat the oven to 300°F. Lightly oil a large baking sheet or spray it with cooking spray. Set aside.
3. In a blender (see Note, page 183), combine the cashews and garlic and process to a paste. Add the nutritional yeast, lemon juice, soy sauce, mustard, and salt and process until well blended. Add as much water as needed, 1 tablespoon at a time, to make a thick sauce.
4. Add the sauce to the kale. Use your fingers to coat the kale completely with the sauce.
5. Arrange the coated kale in a single layer on the prepared baking sheet. Do not allow the leaves to overlap. (If you don't have room for all of the kale, set the remaining leaves aside to bake after the first batch is finished.)

6. Bake the kale leaves for 12 to 15 minutes, then flip them and bake for 5 to 10 minutes longer, watching closely so the kale doesn't burn. When the kale is crisp and dry, remove it from the oven and let cool completely. Kale chips are best when eaten on the same day they are made.

* ***NOTE: If you prefer using dinosaur kale (aka Lacinato or Tuscan kale), the procedure is the same but will require less baking time—usually about 15 minutes total.***

Trail Mix Snack Bites

Makes 16

Like kale chips, snack bars are so easy to make at home that you'll wonder why you ever bought them.

- **1¼ cups old-fashioned rolled oats**
- **1 cup chopped unsalted roasted nuts, any kind or a combination**
- **1 cup raisins, sweetened dried cranberries, chopped pitted dates, other dried fruit, or a combination**
- **½ cup vegan semisweet chocolate chips**
- **½ cup maple syrup**
- **2 tablespoons nut butter, any kind**
- **2 tablespoons vegan butter, such as Earth Balance, melted**
- **1 teaspoon vanilla extract**
- **Water if needed**

1. Preheat the oven to 375°F. Grease an 8-inch square baking pan and set aside.
2. In a food processor, combine the oats, nuts, raisins, and chocolate chips. Process until crumbly. Add the maple syrup, nut butter, vegan butter, and vanilla and process until well combined, adding a little water, a tablespoon at a time, if the mixture is too dry. Press the mixture evenly into the prepared pan.
3. Bake for 20 minutes or until lightly browned. Remove from the oven and set aside to cool. Cover and refrigerate to cool completely before cutting. Cut into 2-inch squares to serve.

Super Slaw

Serves 4

Can you really have a summer barbecue without burgers, beans, and slaw? No, you can't. Slaw is the perfect side dish.

- **¾ cup vegan mayonnaise**
- **¼ cup plain unsweetened nondairy milk, such as soy or almond milk**
- **2 tablespoons fresh lemon juice**
- **1 teaspoon Dijon mustard**
- **1 teaspoon natural sugar, such as Sugar in the Raw**
- **Salt and freshly ground black pepper**
- **1 small head green cabbage, cored and shredded (about 4 cups)**
- **2 carrots, grated**
- **3 red radishes, shredded**
- **2 tablespoons minced scallion**
- **¼ cup raisins or dried cranberries**
- **¼ cup sunflower seeds**

1. In a small bowl, combine the mayonnaise, milk, lemon juice, mustard, sugar, and salt and pepper to taste. Mix until well blended. Set aside.
2. In a large bowl, combine the cabbage, carrots, radishes, scallion, raisins, and sunflower seeds.
3. Add the dressing and toss to mix well. Taste and adjust the seasonings if necessary. Cover and refrigerate. Serve chilled. Store leftovers in a tightly sealed container in the refrigerator for up to 3 days.

Roasted Tomato Bruschette

Serves 4

These bruschette consistently wow vegans and omnivores alike with their simple, potent flavors.

- **1 small red onion, chopped**
- **1 small red bell pepper, seeded and chopped**
- **1 pint cherry or grape tomatoes, halved lengthwise**
- **Extra-virgin olive oil for drizzling and brushing**
- **Salt and freshly ground black pepper**
- **¼ cup minced reconstituted or oil-packed sun-dried tomatoes**
- **¼ cup chopped fresh basil**
- **1 baguette, cut into ½-inch slices**

1. Preheat the oven to 425°F. Lightly oil a shallow 9-by-13-inch baking dish.
2. Combine the onion, bell pepper, and cherry tomatoes in the baking dish. Drizzle with a little olive oil and season with salt and pepper to taste. Roast for 30 minutes or until the vegetables are very soft.
3. Stir the mixture to break up the tomatoes, then stir in the sun-dried tomatoes and basil. Taste and adjust the seasonings if necessary. Set aside and cover loosely to keep warm. Turn the oven to broil.
4. Lightly oil both sides of the bread and arrange on a baking sheet. Broil the bread, turning once until browned on both sides. Be careful not to burn it.
5. To assemble, spoon the hot tomato mixture onto the toasted bread. Serve immediately.

Desserts

Creamy Chocolate Pie

Serves 8

The key to using tofu in desserts is silken tofu—a more custardy variety than what you would use for a stir-fry. Silken tofu is always very soft, as the name implies, but you can use it with recipes calling for tofu of any level of firmness. You can usually find it in the refrigerated section of the grocery store or on the shelves in aseptic packaging.

- **One 12-ounce package silken tofu**
- **One 10-ounce bag vegan semisweet chocolate chips**
- **1 teaspoon vanilla extract**
- **1 premade vegan graham cracker crust**

1. In a blender (see Note, page 183), blend the tofu until smooth.
2. Melt the chocolate chips in the top of a double boiler over hot water or in a microwave, stirring often.
3. When the chocolate is completely melted, add it to the tofu in the blender and process until smooth, then add the vanilla and process again to blend.
4. Pour the filling into the crust and refrigerate until set, about 2 hours. Serve chilled. Store leftover pie in a tightly sealed container in the refrigerator for up to 3 days.

* ***NOTE: The variations on this simple chocolate base are endless. You can line the piecrust with sliced bananas or strawberries, top the filling with fresh raspberries, or add 1/4 cup peanut butter to the filling. Go crazy!***

Chocolate-Almond Truffles

Makes about 24

If you've never made truffles at home before, you'll be surprised by how simple they are to turn out. These rich treats make special occasions significantly more special.

- **8 ounces vegan semisweet chocolate chips**
- **⅓ cup almond butter**
- **⅓ cup confectioners' sugar**
- **2 tablespoons unsweetened almond milk, or as needed**
- **¾ cup slivered almonds, toasted, then finely ground in a food processor**

1. Melt the chocolate in the top of a double boiler over hot water, stirring until smooth. Remove from the heat. Stir in the almond butter until well blended, then add the confectioners' sugar, stirring until smooth and well blended. If the mixture is too dry, stir in the almond milk, 1 tablespoon at a time. Transfer the mixture to a bowl. Cover and refrigerate until firm.

2. Coat the palms of your hands in confectioners' sugar or cocoa. Pinch off about 1½ teaspoons of the mixture and use your hands to shape it into a 1-inch ball. Repeat with the remaining mixture.

3. Roll the truffles in the ground almonds and arrange on a platter or place in small foil or paper candy cups. Enjoy right away or cover and refrigerate for up to 1 week.

Oatmeal Cookies

Makes 24

In the shadow of chocolate chip cookies, oatmeal cookies sometimes play second fiddle. But these subtly spiced, perfectly chewy gems will steal the spotlight.

- **1 cup whole wheat pastry flour or your favorite flour for baking**
- **½ cup natural sugar, such as Sugar in the Raw**
- **1 teaspoon baking soda**
- **1 teaspoon ground cinnamon**
- **½ teaspoon salt**
- **½ cup pure maple syrup**
- **¼ cup applesauce**
- **1½ teaspoons vanilla extract**
- **1¾ cups old-fashioned rolled oats**

1. Preheat the oven to 350°F. Lightly grease one or two baking sheets or line them with parchment paper and set aside.
2. Combine the flour, sugar, baking soda, cinnamon, and salt in a large bowl and set aside.
3. In a small bowl, combine the maple syrup, applesauce, and vanilla and mix well. Combine the wet ingredients with the dry ingredients, stirring to mix. Stir in the oats until well combined.
4. Drop the dough by the heaping tablespoonful about 2 inches apart onto the prepared baking sheet. Flatten the cookies with your fingers or the back of the spoon.
5. Bake on the center rack for 12 to 14 minutes, until the cookies are lightly browned on the bottom. (If using two pans, you can bake them one at a time or put one pan on the bottom rack and rotate the pans halfway through the baking time.) Remove from the oven and let cool on a rack for a few minutes. Cool completely before storing in an airtight container at room temperature for up to 5 days.

Old-Fashioned Apple Crisp

Serves 8

Cinnamon, sugar, and a crumbly topping combine to make a showstopping dairy-free dessert. Top with a scoop of vegan vanilla ice cream.

- **4 to 5 Granny Smith or other cooking apples, peeled, cored, and sliced**
- **¼ cup plus 1 tablespoon unbleached all-purpose flour**
- **¾ cup natural sugar, such as Sugar in the Raw**
- **1 tablespoon fresh lemon juice**
- **1½ teaspoons ground cinnamon**
- **1 cup old-fashioned rolled oats**
- **3 tablespoons vegan butter, such as Earth Balance, softened**

1. Preheat the oven to 375°F. Lightly grease an 8-inch square baking dish or spray it with cooking spray and set aside.
2. In a large bowl, combine the apples, 1 tablespoon of the flour, ½ cup of the sugar, the lemon juice, and ½ teaspoon of the cinnamon. Mix gently, transfer to the prepared dish, and set aside.
3. In a small bowl, combine the oats, the remaining ¼ cup flour, the remaining ¼ cup sugar, the remaining 1 teaspoon cinnamon, and the vegan butter. Mix with your hands to combine thoroughly.
4. Sprinkle the topping over the apple mixture. Bake for about 35 minutes, until the fruit bubbles in the center and the topping is nicely browned. Serve warm. Tightly wrap any leftover crisp and store in the refrigerator for up to 3 days.

Coconut Cupcakes

Makes 12

These cupcakes are a coconut triple threat. Coconut milk is used in the cake batter, coconut extract adds flavor to the frosting, and shredded coconut makes decorating these tropical treats extra easy.

FOR THE CUPCAKES

- **¾ cup unsweetened coconut milk (see Note, page 163)**
- **1½ teaspoons cider vinegar**
- **1¼ cups unbleached all-purpose flour or whole wheat pastry flour**
- **½ cup unsweetened shredded dried coconut**
- **1 teaspoon baking powder**
- **¼ teaspoon baking soda**
- **¼ teaspoon salt**
- **¾ cup natural sugar, such as Sugar in the Raw**
- **⅓ cup neutral-flavored vegetable oil**
- **1 teaspoon coconut extract**

FOR THE FROSTING

- **1 cup vegan butter, such as Earth Balance**
- **4 cups confectioners' sugar**
- **2 tablespoons unsweetened coconut milk**
- **1 teaspoon coconut extract**
- **1 cup unsweetened shredded dried coconut**

1. Preheat the oven to 350°F. Line a 12-cup muffin tin with cupcake liners. Set aside.
2. To make the cupcakes, combine the ¾ cup coconut milk and the vinegar in a small bowl. Set aside.
3. In a medium bowl, combine the flour, ½ cup coconut, baking powder, baking soda, and salt. Mix to combine.
4. In a large bowl, combine the sugar, oil, and coconut extract. Stir in the coconut milk mixture. Add the dry ingredients to the wet ingredients and stir until smooth.

5. Pour the batter evenly into the prepared tin, filling the cups about two-thirds full, and bake for about 20 minutes, until a toothpick inserted in the center of a cupcake comes out clean. Let cool completely before frosting.

6. While the cupcakes are baking, make the frosting. In a large bowl, cream the vegan butter with an electric mixer on high speed until light and fluffy. Add the confectioners' sugar, 2 tablespoons coconut milk, and 1 teaspoon coconut extract. Mix until thoroughly blended. Continue mixing for about 2 minutes until the frosting is smooth and stiff.

7. When the cupcakes are completely cool, top them with the frosting. Place the 1 cup shredded coconut on a plate and dip the frosted top of each cupcake into it. Store leftover cupcakes in a tightly sealed container in the refrigerator for up to 5 days.

Pumpkin Cheesecake

Serves 8

Even the traditionally dairy-rich cheesecake can be made vegan. A blend of tofu and vegan cream cheese ensures that the cake is fluffy and rich all at once. The extra spice of gingersnap cookies in the crust elevates this fall favorite and makes it a spectacular dish for an autumn dinner party.

FOR THE CRUST

- **1½ cups vegan graham cracker crumbs or gingersnap crumbs**
- **4 tablespoons vegan butter, such as Earth Balance, melted**

FOR THE FILLING

- **Two 8-ounce packages vegan cream cheese**
- **One 12-ounce package firm silken tofu**
- **One 16-ounce can solid-pack pumpkin puree**
- **¾ cup natural sugar, such as Sugar in the Raw**
- **¼ cup maple syrup**
- **2 tablespoons cornstarch**
- **1¼ teaspoons ground cinnamon**
- **¼ teaspoon ground allspice**
- **¼ teaspoon freshly grated nutmeg**
- **¼ teaspoon ground ginger**

1. Preheat the oven to 350°F. Lightly oil a 9-inch springform pan or coat it with nonstick cooking spray. Place the crumbs in the pan, add the melted vegan butter, and toss with a fork to combine. Press the crumb mixture into the bottom and sides of the pan and bake for 5 minutes. Remove from the oven, leaving the oven on, and set aside to cool.
2. In a food processor, combine the cream cheese and tofu and process until smooth and blended. Add the pumpkin, sugar, maple syrup, cornstarch, cinnamon, allspice, nutmeg, and ginger. Process until thoroughly combined and well blended, stopping to scrape down the sides of the processor as needed.

3. Spread the filling evenly into the cooled crust. Bake for 45 minutes or until firm. Turn off the oven and allow the cheesecake to remain in the oven for 15 minutes longer.
4. Remove from the oven and allow to cool completely at room temperature. Refrigerate for several hours before serving. To serve, run a thin knife around the perimeter of the cake to loosen it from the springform pan, then release and remove the sides of the pan and slice the cheesecake. Tightly cover any leftover cheesecake and refrigerate for up to 3 days.

Easy Ice Cream Cake

Serves 8

A deceptively easy dessert, this ice cream cake looks like it takes hours to make but comes together in minutes (not including freezing time). Mix up the sorbet flavor and toppings to fit the rest of your menu or tastes. Birthdays will never be the same after you've tried this treat.

- **1½ cups vegan chocolate cookie crumbs**
- **¼ cup vegan butter, such as Earth Balance, melted**
- **1 pint vegan vanilla ice cream, softened**
- **1 pint raspberry sorbet, softened**
- **Chocolate curls**
- **Fresh raspberries**

1. Preheat the oven to 350°F. Lightly oil an 8-inch springform pan or coat it with nonstick cooking spray. Put the cookie crumbs and melted butter in the prepared pan and mix well to combine. Press the crumb mixture onto the bottom and sides of the pan. Bake for 5 minutes, then allow to cool.

2. Place the softened ice cream in a large bowl, stirring until smooth. Add the softened sorbet and use a spoon to streak it throughout the ice cream. Scrape the ice cream mixture evenly into the prepared crust, smoothing the top. Freeze for several hours or overnight.

3. Before serving, bring the cake to room temperature for 5 minutes, then carefully remove the sides of the pan. Sprinkle chocolate curls on top of the cake around the outside and pile berries in the center. Serve immediately. Tightly wrapped, leftover cake will keep well in the freezer for up to 2 weeks.

Chocolate Chip Cookies

Makes about 36

Baking without eggs is a cinch once you get a few basics down. The applesauce in these indulgent cookies replaces the egg and adds a small boost of nutrition. Serve chocolate chip cookies with (nondairy) milk, of course.

- **2 cups whole wheat pastry flour**
- **½ teaspoon baking powder**
- **½ teaspoon baking soda**
- **¼ teaspoon salt**
- **½ cup natural sugar, such as Sugar in the Raw**
- **⅓ cup maple syrup**
- **⅓ cup applesauce**
- **3 tablespoons nondairy milk, such as soy or almond milk**
- **1 teaspoon vanilla extract**
- **1½ cups vegan semisweet chocolate chips (see Note)**

1. Preheat the oven to 350°F. Lightly oil two baking sheets.
2. In a medium bowl, combine the flour, baking powder, baking soda, and salt. Set aside.
3. In a large bowl, combine the sugar, maple syrup, applesauce, nondairy milk, and vanilla. Stir until well blended. Add the dry ingredients to the wet ingredients and mix until just combined. Fold in the chocolate chips.
4. Drop the dough by the tablespoonful onto the prepared baking sheets, about 2 inches apart.
5. Bake on the center rack for 15 to 18 minutes, until lightly browned on the bottom. (If using two pans, you can bake them one at a time or put one pan on the bottom rack and rotate the pans halfway through.) Let cool completely before storing in an airtight container at room temperature for up to 1 week.

* ***NOTE: Look for vegan brand semisweet chocolate chips at stores like Whole Foods and Trader Joe's. Some brands are "accidentally" vegan. For example, Ghirardelli semisweet chocolate chips and those by Guittard have no butterfat and are thus vegan. Be sure to check the labels.***

Fabulous Fudgy Brownies

Makes 9

Even vegans need brownies. Whether you top them with nondairy ice cream or whipped cream or eat them straight from the oven, these brownies are fudgy and rich and satisfying.

- **½ cup applesauce**
- **¼ cup pure maple syrup**
- **¼ cup unsweetened almond milk**
- **3 tablespoons neutral-flavored vegetable oil**
- **1½ teaspoons vanilla extract**
- **1 cup all-purpose flour**
- **½ cup natural sugar, such as Sugar in the Raw**
- **⅓ cup unsweetened cocoa powder**
- **1½ teaspoons baking powder**
- **1 tablespoon instant coffee or espresso granules (optional; see Note)**
- **¼ teaspoon salt**
- **⅔ cup vegan semisweet chocolate chips**
- **½ cup chopped walnuts or pecans (optional)**

1. Preheat the oven to 350°F. Lightly grease an 8-inch square baking pan or spray it with cooking spray.
2. Combine the applesauce, maple syrup, almond milk, oil, and vanilla in a large bowl. Stir to mix well.
3. In a separate bowl, combine the flour, sugar, cocoa, baking powder, coffee, and salt. Mix well.
4. Use a rubber spatula to stir the dry ingredients into the wet mixture until just combined. Do not overmix. Fold in the chocolate chips and walnuts.

5. Scrape the batter into the pan and spread it evenly. Bake for 30 minutes or until a toothpick inserted in the center comes out almost clean. Let the brownies cool completely in the pan before cutting into squares. Store tightly covered in the refrigerator for up to 1 week or freeze for 1 to 2 months.

* ***NOTE: The optional instant coffee or espresso granules deepen the chocolate flavor in the brownies.***

RESOURCES

MAGAZINES

Chickpea (chickpeamagazine.com)
Laika (laikamagazine.com)
Vegan Health & Fitness (veganhealthandfitnessmag.com)
VegNews (vegnews.com)

BOOKS

Becoming Vegan, Brenda Davis and Vesanto Melina
Beg, Rory Freedman
Crazy Sexy Diet, Kris Carr
Eating Animals, Jonathan Safran Foer
The Everything Vegan Pregnancy Book, Reed Mangels
The Face on Your Plate, Jeffrey Moussaief Masson
Finding Ultra, Rich Roll
The Jungle, Upton Sinclair
The Kind Life, Alicia Silverstone
The Lean, Kathy Freston
Mad Cowboy, Howard F. Lyman with Glen Merzer
Thrive, Brendan Brazier
VB6, Mark Bittman
Vegan for Life, Jack Norris and Virginia Messina
Vegan Pregnancy Survival Guide, Sayward Rebhal

COOKBOOKS

Artisan Vegan Cheese, Miyoko Schinner
Celebrate Vegan, Dynise Balcavage
Chloe's Kitchen, Chloe Coscarelli
The Conscious Cook, Tal Ronnen
Crazy Sexy Kitchen, Kris Carr and Chad Sarno

Gluten-Free and Vegan Holidays, Jennifer Katzinger
Grilling Vegan Style, John Schlimm
The Inspired Vegan, Bryant Terry
Isa Does It, Isa Chandra Moskowitz
1,000 Vegan Recipes, Robin Robertson
Plum, Makini Howell
Quick Fix Vegan, Robin Robertson
The Sexy Vegan Cookbook, Brian Patton
Spork-Fed, Jenny Engel and Heather Goldberg
Vegan Cooking for Carnivores, Roberto Martin
Vegan Eats World, Terry Hope Romero
Vegan Holiday Kitchen, Nava Atlas
Veganomicon, Terry Hope Romero and Isa Chandra Moskowitz
Vegan Sandwiches Save the Day, Celine Steen and Tamasin Noyes

ORGANIZATIONS

Compassion over Killing (cok.net)
The Environmental Working Group (ewg.org)
The Humane Society of the United States (hsus.org)
International Vegetarian Union (ivu.org)
Meatless Monday (meatlessmonday.com)
Mercy for Animals (mercyforanimals.org)
People for the Ethical Treatment of Animals (peta.org)
Physicians Committee for Responsible Medicine (pcrm.org)
The Vegan Society (vegansociety.com)
Vegetarian Resource Group (vrg.org)

RESTAURANTS

Boston

Grasshopper Restaurant (grasshoppervegan.com)
My Thai Vegan Café and Bubble Tea Bistro
Red Lentil (theredlentil.com)

Chicago

The Chicago Diner (veggiediner.com)
Karyn's on Green (karynsongreen.com)
Native Foods Café (nativefoods.com)
Upton's Breakroom (uptonsnaturals.com/breakroom)

Las Vegas

Wynn and Encore restaurants (wynnlasvegas.com/restaurants)
Ronald's Donuts (yelp.com/biz/ronalds-donuts-las-vegas)

Los Angeles

Crossroads Kitchen (crossroadskitchen.com)
M Café (mcafedechaya.com)
Shojin (theshojin.com)

New York City

Atlas Café (atlascafenyc.com)
Blythe Ann's
Candle 79 (candle79.com)
Champs (champsdiner.com)
'sNice (snicecafe.com)

Philadelphia

Blackbird Pizzeria (blackbirdpizzeria.com)
HipCityVeg (hipcityveg.com)
Vedge (facebook.com/pages/Vedge-Restaurant/233351833356847)

Portland, Oregon

Homegrown Smoker Vegan BBQ (homegrownsmoker.wordpress.com)
Portobello (portobellopdx.com)

San Francisco

Gracias Madre (gracias-madre.com)
Ike's Place (ilikeikesplace.com)
Millennium (millenniumrestaurant.com)

Washington, D.C.

Great Sage (greatsage.com)
Sticky Fingers (stickyfingersbakery.com)
Woodland's Vegan Bistro (woodlandsveganbistro.net)

SANCTUARIES

Farm Sanctuary (farmsanctuary.org)
The Gentle Barn (gentlebarn.org)
Woodstock Farm Animal Sanctuary (woodstocksanctuary.org)

TRAVEL

Deer Run Bed & Breakfast
Big Pine Key, Florida
deerrunfloridabb.com

El Remanso Lodge
Puerto Jimenez, Costa Rica
elremanso.com

The Farm
Lipa City, Philippines
thefarm.com.ph

Five Elements
Mambal, Bali, Indonesia
fivelements.org/en

The Ginger Cat Bed & Breakfast
Rock Stream, New York
gingercat-bb.com

Haramara Retreat
Sayulita, Mexico
haramararetreat.com

Holistic Holiday at Sea
atasteofhealth.org

The Stanford Inn
Mendocino, California
stanfordinn.com

Ten Thousand Waves
Santa Fe, New Mexico
tenthousandwaves.com

Tierno Tours
tiernotours.com

Vegan mini-mall (Herbivore Clothing Company, Scapegoat Tattoo, Food Fight Grocery, and Sweetpea Baking Company)
Portland, Oregon
herbivoreclothing.com
scapegoattattoo.com
foodfightgrocery.com
sweetpeabaking.com

VegVoyages
vegvoyages.com

Wynn and Encore
Las Vegas, Nevada
wynnlasvegas.com

OTHER RESOURCES

Barnivore (barnivore.com)
Happy Cow (happycow.net)
Nutrition Data (nutritiondata.self.com)
Rose Pedals Vegan Weddings (rosepedalsveganweddings.com)

ACKNOWLEDGMENTS

Getting to write this book was a dream come true. I'll be eternally grateful to Lia Ronnen for giving me this incredible opportunity, to Judy Pray for giving me the idea and making it work and answering a zillion inane first-time-author questions, and to the entire team at Artisan. Without the phenomenally good recipes of Robin Robertson, the book would have ended with a shrug and a plate of raw kale.

My years as a professional vegan would not have been possible without Colleen Holland, a friend and mentor. They also brought the utter delight of knowing my BBTCBs, Sutton Long, Jennifer Chen, Anna Peraino, and Hilary Pollack. There are friends without whom nothing, much less this book, would have been possible. Thank you to Bekah Brunstetter, Arthur Combs, Joelle Schwartz, Margaret Widlund, Santiago Perry, and Peter Ryan for being. It's an honor to know and work with the likes of Leanne Mai-ly Hilgart, Joshua Katcher, Tal Ronnen, Chris Kerr, Corinne Bowen, Kris Carr, Ben Adams, and Paul Shapiro, among many, many others.

There is no way to properly thank my family in words for how wonderful they are. Louie, Susy, Sheila, Kevin, and Mason Danger are the best family members anyone could ask for, and I'm in constant, grateful disbelief that they're mine.

A mi querido Ricardo, muchísimas gracias. Hay dos epocas en mi vida: antes que llegaste, y después. Te adoro.

INDEX

Note: Page numbers in *italics* refer to illustrations.

M

N

O

P

Q

R

S

T

U

V